SlowItDownCKD 2016

When my family doctor told me I probably had a problem and it had to do with my kidneys, maybe Chronic Kidney Disease, my first reaction was to demand in no uncertain terms, "What Is It and How Did I Get It?" Hence, the title of my first CKD book.

There are many, many of us out there. By us, I mean those who have Chronic Kidney Disease. Friends and family of CKD patients can also gain some insight into the daily travails of living with the disease via this book of 2016's *SlowItDownCKD* blogs. I am no expert, but I have read just about every book concerning this problem that I could find. Of course, most medical texts are not included because I couldn't understand them. Most of the kidney disease cookbooks aren't included because I can understand a heavy duty medical text better than I can a cookbook. I even read memoirs and biographies to glean what information I could...and I researched, researched, researched.

Surprisingly, very few of these books dealt with the early or moderate stages of the disease. These are the stages when we, as patients, are most shocked, confused, and possibly depressed. I didn't want to read about transplants or kidney failure. They scared me and I just wasn't ready to learn about them yet.

But I did want to know what was happening to me on a daily basis, what the medications that were ordered for me were supposed to do, and what new discoveries there were that might help slow down this deterioration of my kidneys. That's what this collection of 2016's blogs is about.

The more you know about Chronic Kidney Disease and the more anecdotes you read about other people's relationship with it, the more comfortable you'll feel in the early or moderate stages of having the disease yourself. I sure wish someone had blogged about it when it was new to me.

I've discovered I have 17,000 readers in 106 countries and they're not afraid to tell me what they need to know. I research for them and respond with a blog post, but remind them they need to speak with their nephrologist and/or renal nutritionist before taking any action. And I repeatedly remind my readers that I am not a doctor.

I've written four previous books about Chronic Kidney Disease that you'll find referenced many times in the blogs. Those books are *What Is It and How Did I Get It? Early Stage Chronic Kidney Disease*; *The Book of Blogs: Moderate Stage Chronic Kidney Disease, Part 1*; *The Book of Blogs: Moderate Stage Chronic Kidney Disease, Part 2*; and *SlowItDownCKD 2015*.

I started blogging after a doctor in India contacted me telling me he wanted his patients to have the first book, but sometimes they couldn't even afford the bus fare to the clinic. I suggested I start the blog (not having a clue how to do that), he translate it, then print it and give it to his patients. The idea was that those who could make it to the clinic would bring the printed copies of the blog back to their communities. This is one of the most rewarding services I've ever performed.

In the interest of keeping this book from becoming mammoth, I've removed the pictures, diagrams, and news of past events. I also removed my signature closing: "Until next week, keep living your life!" After all, how many times can you read the same sentence in a single book? URLs have been removed, too, since you can't very well click through in a print book.

Welcome to *SlowItDownCKD 2016*.

Keep living your life!

Gail

p.s. I want Bear to know how much I STILL appreciate his respecting Monday as blog day, and when I'm writing a book, Monday, Tuesday, Wednesday, Thursday, Friday, Saturday, and Sunday as writing days. You're one of a kind, honey.

1/4/16 *Electronically Speaking*

Happy New Year to each and every one of you. I've been looking at quite a few CKD pages on Facebook and was, once again, reminded how quickly things change. Only one of the three pages I listed in 2011's *What Is It and How Did I Get It? Early Stage Chronic Kidney Disease* is still in existence.

That's *The Transplant Community Outreach* with 5,897 members which is "... an online support group of individuals and families who are recipients, are waiting for a transplant, are donor family members, caregivers, or those who have a connection with organ donation and transplantation." I like that they've asked me to post this blog weekly, although it is about moderate stage chronic kidney disease.

I offered another list of such pages in *The Book of Blogs: Moderate Stage Chronic Kidney Disease, Part 2* which was published only last year.

- *Kidney Disease and Diet Ideas and Help 1*

- *Show Your Scars Tour*

- *Kidney Disease Is Not a Joke*

- *The Transplant Community Outreach* {I write *Kidney Matters* for them at their request.}

- *Renal Patient Support Group*

- *Chronic Kidney Disease*

- *P2P {Peer To Peer}*

- *But You Don't Look Sick*

- *TCO Women's Health*

- *Kidney Disease Shout Board*

To the best of my knowledge, *Show Your Scars Tour, Chronic Kidney Disease,* and *TCO Women's Health* are no longer with us. But, there are loads of additional pages for us, including some secret groups that I don't think I'm at liberty to write about. Comment if you'd like to know more about secret groups and I will gladly contact the administrator of the appropriate one for you. Some of the other pages I read are:

- *Kidney Advocates* which is a brand new page administrated by the ever striving advocate, James Myers. This man has invited me to post the blog on every page he's involved with. If it's possible, he may be more serious about advocacy than I am.

- *Kidney Disease Ideas and Diet 1* (not to be confused with *Kidney Disease and Diet Ideas and Help 1)* whose former administrator has become an online friend since we share so many of the same issues in our personal lives. The purpose of this page is simple: "...Sometimes in life we need a little hand up. Battling kidney disease and getting new dietary instruction can be hard. Every stage is different. We are here to help."

- *Stage 3 'n 4 CKD Kidneybeaners Gathering Place*, a smaller, highly active group moderated by my favorite wisenheimer, Robin Rose, who – as a lay person – has an incredible understanding of medicalese. As she writes, "Stage 3 'n 4 CKD is a unique place to live – predialysis medicine isn't that available… so we gather together to share, to support, to learn, to research, and to thrive together… speak your story, your experience, your feelings, your research… let's commit to staying healthy together!"

- *Women's Renal Failure Support Group* which is fast becoming a favorite since I can be a bit of a prude, but this is women only (as they have to keep reminding men who try to post on the page).

These are some I'm active on are (in alphabetical order):

British Kidney Patient Association

Chronic Kidney Disease Support Group

Dialysis & Kidney Disease

GM Kidney Information Network

I Hate Dialysis

Kidney disease isn't for sissies

Kidney Disease, Dialysis, and Transplant

MANI TRUST

People on dialysis

Renal Patient Support Group

There's even a page for the buying and selling of Chronic Disease paraphernalia which is called, appropriately enough, *P2P's Chronic Illness Awareness Buy & Sell* and administered by Sandie Jones who is also the administrator of Peer to Peer (P2P). That's no surprise, but it is innovative.

And last, but not least, we have (ahem) *SlowItDownCKD* where I post Chronic Kidney Disease related medical tidbits that I've found by perusing different medical sites, Twitter, Instagram, Pinterest, newspapers, medical journals, even medical texts. I am limited as to what I post since I've made it a firm policy to post only what I understand. Whoops, there go the CKD diet cookbooks right out the window.

These posts also appear on Twitter as @SlowItDownCKD. I have found some really CKD informative people or organizations to follow there. My all-time favorite is @kidney_boy, nephrologist Joel Topf, who answers my questions and includes me in as much nephrology work as he can considering I'm a layman. Lay woman?

Same for @nephondemand (Dr. Tejas Desai) who also answers whatever I ask. I also follow nurses, doctors, teaching institutions, renal dieticians, anyone who is some way connected to CKD.

I am surprised every time a doctor, nurse, teaching institution, or renal dietician follows me. I make it very clear that I am NOT a doctor, just a layman (Oh, here we go again: lay woman?) who has Chronic Kidney Disease and wants to make certain everyone everywhere in the whole wide world is aware of its existence so they'll get tested.

Here's hoping 2016 is, indeed, Sweet 16 for you. There's nothing wrong with making each new year the best year you've had yet. Gratitude and service are the way to go in my book (Yep, I'm punning.)

1/11/16 *To Wash or Not To Wash*

I was thinking about language when I took a shower last night. Then the bottle of shampoo I was using caught my eye. It had the words 'sulfate free' in large letters on the label. Hmmm, sulfate looked a lot like sulphur. Were they related?

After checking a bunch of dictionaries, I decided to use the definition of The Medical Dictionary since it seemed the simplest to understand: "a salt of sulfuric acid"

Uh-oh, sulfuric means made of sulfur. Although the spelling may be different, sulfuric acid is highly corrosive. It's also a mineral... and is used in both waste water treatment and fertilizer creation. Why would shampoo have this ingredient in the first place?

I figured the best person to provide an answer would be a hair stylist, so I read Melissa Jongman's article "Sulfates: Are they damaging your hair? Why to opt for a sulfate free shampoo.

"Sulfates are detergents used to make the shampoo lather. They're inexpensive to use in shampoos, which explains why more than 90% of shampoos contain them. The most common sulfates used in these shampoos are:

- Sodium Lauryl Sulphate (SLS)

- Sodium Laureth Sulphate (SLES)

- Ammonia Laureth Sulphate (ALS)

- TEA Lauryeth Sulfate (TEA)

- Sodium Myreth Sulphate (SMS)"

This was not looking good. Sulphur is something we, as Chronic Kidney Disease patients, need to avoid. As I explained in *What Is It and How Did I Get It? Early Stage Chronic Kidney Disease,* sulphur can further damage your already damaged kidneys. So what can we do? Not washing our hair is obviously not the answer. I googled shampoos without sulfates and came up with a list of 43 from sulfatefreeshampoos.org. While the latest edit of this list was during this new year, I am not familiar with the editors nor the products. However, you can safely bet that I'll try them.

Let's go back to why sulfates are not good for CKD patients for a minute. I stumbled across a CKD education site called quizlet.com. Perusing this site, I found the statement "Very late CKD is due to reduced excretion of sulfates and phosphates."

Of course! That makes perfect sense: as our kidney function declines, we are not excreting as much of these substances as we did before we were lucky enough (ouch!) to develop CKD and they build up. That's CKD 101.

A nervous me decided to see what other beauty or health products used sulfates. I discovered it's used in body wash (Wait! Isn't sulfate a skin irritant?), tooth-paste, and nail polish. That tripped a thought. Didn't I blog about that?

I used the search function on the blog only to find that that blog dealt with other chemicals in nail polish. (Gritting teeth and crying out in anguish) Is nothing safe anymore? All right, pick a chemical... any chemical.

Looking at the ingredients in both hair products and nail polish, I chose phthalates. The Centers for Disease Control and Prevention (CDC) helped us out with this one:

"Phthalates are a group of chemicals used to make plastics more flexible and harder to break. ... They are used in hundreds of products, such as vinyl flooring, adhesives, detergents, lubricating oils, automotive plastics, plastic clothes (raincoats), and personal care products (soaps, shampoos, hair sprays, and nail polishes)....

How Phthalates Affect People's Health

Human health effects from exposure to low levels of phthalates are unknown. Some types of phthalates have affected the reproductive system of laboratory animals. More research is needed to assess the human health effects of exposure to phthalates."

Maybe the human health effects are unknown and maybe this passes quickly via the urine, but if you have Chronic Kidney Disease, you are not filtering your blood as well as other people. Why take a chance of making it worse?

Now that I've probably made you fearful of using any beauty product on the market, be aware that there are many products without phthalate. Breast Cancer Action (Yes, there seems to be a connection between breast cancer and phthalates.) offers a list of companies which produce phthalate free beauty aids.

Let's talk about service and gratitude for just a minute. While I've always believed in service, it's only since I've been diagnosed with Chronic Kidney Disease (way back in in 2008) that I've become aware of how very thankful I am for the little things in life – like spreading CKD Awareness by writing this blog, posting some CKD tidbit on Twitter daily, starting an Instagram account for *SlowItDownCKD*, and offering my books. Thank YOU for being the readers.

1/18/16 *Another Cause of CKD?*

I love it when my friends look out for me. And I, in turn, want to look out for you. That's why I'll be writing about a problem my friends made certain I was aware of today. Let's go way back to the beginning for this one.

I had had something: heartburn, upset stomach, acid reflux??? a few months ago. Not having experienced digestive problems before I didn't know what it was. Heck, I didn't even know if it was a digestive problem, but I knew I couldn't take the nausea and sensitive stomach too much longer without investigating. After weeks of this not going away on its own, I made an appointment with my trusted primary care doctor.

While I was waiting for the appointment, I took a look at *Medical Surgical Nursing: Critical Thinking for Collaborative Care, 4th Ed.* although I can only understand some of it and we know how dangerous a little knowledge can be. According to what I read, it didn't seem that I had an ulcer. Hmmm, maybe gastritis?

Something seemed off with what I was reading, sort of out of sync, so I checked copyright date. Uh huh, the book is 14 years old… and outdated. Time for a newer edition. Case in point and message sent: check the copyright dates of any medical texts you have. They get outdated fast these days.

Okay, let's see what the doctor had to say. She addressed my 'abdominal pain in the pit of my stomach' and the nausea, diagnosing it as 'epigastric pain' and nausea. Well, how is that different from stomach pain?

The stomach is defined by WebMD in this way:

"The stomach is a muscular organ located on the left side of the upper abdomen. The stomach receives food from the esophagus. As food reaches the end of the esophagus, it enters the stomach through a muscular valve called the lower esophageal sphincter.

The stomach secretes acid and enzymes that digest food. Ridges of muscle tissue called rugae line the stomach. The stomach muscles contract periodically, churning food to enhance digestion. The pyloric sphincter is a muscular valve that opens to allow food to pass from the stomach to the small intestine."

I always get the stomach and the abdomen mixed up, so I looked that up too. Healthline was helpful here.

"The abdomen is the area below the chest and above the pelvis. It is comprised of muscles, vertebrae, ribs, blood vessels, nerves, and several vital organs, including the liver, small intestine, large intestine, and kidneys."

Oh, so the stomach is part of the abdomen.

We still need one more definition here: Epigastric. According to The Free Dictionary, that means, "The upper middle region of the abdomen." Ah, another part of the abdomen.

The good doctor prescribed 40 mg. of Omeprazole each morning before breakfast. Omeprazole's generic name is Prilosec. I saw nothing in the pharmacy handout for this medication that related specifically to CKD.

However, the risk doesn't seem to be to me since I already have CKD but to those who use these drugs who do not yet have CKD. I do wonder if it could cause Acute Kidney Injury or acute interstitial nephritis (both short term as opposed to chronic) in those who both already suffer from CKD and use these drugs since it's not made clear in the articles.

There are many versions of this announcement but I'll be using the one from HealthDay since it is the least medicalese one I've located.

"MONDAY, Jan. 11, 2016 (HealthDay News) — A type of heartburn medication called proton pump inhibitors may be linked to long-term kidney damage, a new study suggests.

Prilosec, Nexium and Prevacid belong to this class of drugs, which treat heartburn and acid reflux by lowering the amount of acid produced by the stomach.

People who use proton pump inhibitors (PPIs) have a 20 percent to 50 percent higher risk of chronic kidney disease compared with nonusers, said lead author Dr. Morgan Grams, an assistant professor of epidemiology at Johns Hopkins University in Baltimore.

The study was published Jan. 11 in *JAMA Internal Medicine*.

The study doesn't establish a direct cause-and-effect relationship between the drugs and chronic kidney disease. However, Grams said, 'We found there was an increasing risk associated with an increasing dose. That suggests that perhaps this observed effect is real.'"

This information is brand, spanking new. I would suggest speaking to your doctor if you are taking one of these medications. I would not suggest doing anything – such as stopping without medical advice – in a panic. I'm a nut about my health and even I spoke this over with my PCP, who I might mention, is a highly collaborative doctor, one who listens to what I have to say and talks it over with me. Now that's the way to have a doctor.

1/25/16 *Good Enough*

Yesterday, I carefully applied my eye liner, examined myself in the magnifying mirror, nodded to myself and murmured, "Good enough." I've been saying that an awful lot lately and finally realized – once a valued, constant reader asked about the connection between worsening vision and Chronic Kidney Disease – that it may be due to my CKD.

This, after I've spent years attributing "Good enough" to the slowest developing ever case of macular degeneration, the age related need for reading glasses, and my impatience with makeup. Of course, then I remembered that I couldn't read a darned thing without the reading glasses and, that without ample light, even they didn't do the trick.

Back to the drawing board, ladies and gentlemen. Here's what DaVita has to say about CKD and vision.

"Diabetes and high blood pressure aren't only the leading causes of chronic kidney disease (CKD). They're also the leading causes of eye disease and loss of vision. If your renal disease is a result of either condition your vision may be at risk.

Some of the most common eye problems that occur in CKD patients are retinopathy, cataracts and glaucoma."

Here are some quickie reminders before we continue.

The American Diabetes Association tells us, "Diabetes is a group of diseases characterized by high blood glucose levels that result from defects in the body's ability to produce and/or use insulin."

I turned to *What Is It and How Did I Get It? Early Stage Chronic Kidney* for a reminder about high blood pressure: "A possible cause of CKD, 140/90mm Hg is currently considered hypertension, a risk factor for heart disease and stroke, too."

However, the American Heart Association has changed this a bit as of Dec. 2013. "The American Heart Association maintains its recommendation of initiating treatment — starting with lifestyle changes and then medication if necessary — at 140/90 until age 80, then at 150/90." Yet, *The Journal of the American Medical Association* maintains that people over 60 should not be considered hypertensive until they register 150/90.

While that's not new information to me, I did wonder how hypertension could affect your sight. The American Academy of Ophthalmology came to the rescue here.

"If the blood pressure is very high it can be called malignant hypertension and cause swelling of the macula and acute loss of vision. Otherwise hypertension can cause progressive constriction of the arterioles in the eye and other findings. Usually high blood pressure alone will not affect vision much, however hypertension is a known risk factor in the onset and/or progression of other eye disease such as glaucoma, diabetic retinopathy, and macular degeneration as well as blocked veins and arteries in the retina or nerve of the eye that can severely affect vision."

My first response to this information was, "What's an arteriole? A small artery?" Time to find out. I turned to my old friend MedicineNet for the definition: "A small branch of an artery that leads to a capillary. The oxygenated hemoglobin (oxyhemoglobin) makes the blood in arterioles (and arteries) look bright red."

That makes sense. Do you remember what glaucoma and/or macular degeneration are? Back to another trusted source for one of the definitions: The Mayo Clinic.

"Glaucoma is a group of eye conditions that damage the optic nerve, which is vital to good vision. This damage is often caused by an abnormally high pressure in your eye."

I sort of, maybe, remembered writing about macular generation in *The Book of Blogs: Moderate Stage Chronic Kidney Disease, Part 2*. Sure enough, I found it.

"An eye disease that progressively destroys the macula, the central portion of the retina, impairing central vision. Macular degeneration rarely causes total blindness because only the center of vision is affected." Oh, MedicineNet again. That's a good source for easily understood medical definitions if you're looking for one.

Let's say you don't have diabetes or hypertension. Does CKD affect your vision then? Interestingly enough, most sites I pulled up talked more about CKD being caught during an eye exam than CKD causing vision problems... except in diabetic End Stage Renal Disease. This is when you need to have your eyes carefully checked and often.

PubMed, part of the US National Library of Medicine, National Institutes of Health, puts a bit of a different spin on the vision/CKD exploration. "Retinal abnormalities are common in inherited and acquired renal disease."

Wow! This is from an older study – 2011 – conducted by the well-respected *Clinical Journal of the American Society of Nephrology*. I don't know if my CKD is inherited or acquired, but it is renal disease and I do have vision problems... and so does one of my valued, constant readers.

By the way, blurred vision may be an indication that you are suffering from uremia. This reminder brought to you by the Renal Network's Kidney Patient News.

Of course, I can almost hear some of you asking what uremia is. *The Book of Blogs: Moderate Stage Chronic Kidney Disease, Part 1* was of help here: it's "the buildup of waste in the blood due to kidney failure."

I really enjoy learning from the research I do to answer your questions, so thank you for another opportunity to do that. Just keep in mind that I'm not a doctor and you need to ask these questions of your nephrologist who will answer them or refer you to another specialist if need be.

2/1/16 *Damned If You Do and Damned If You Don't*

It is absolutely amazing how many things can go wrong with the human body. Some, such as cancer, are drastic while others, like a general feeling of being unwell or fatigue (sound familiar, Chronic Kidney Disease sufferers?), are not. For example, Bear has developed the Helicobacter pylori infection. This, according to MedlinePlus (part of the U.S. National Library of Medicine) is

"… a type of bacteria that causes infection in the stomach. It is found in about two-thirds of the world's population. It may be spread by unclean food and water, but researchers aren't sure. It causes Peptic ulcers and can also cause stomach cancer."

That made me nervous. I immediately (and unfairly) blamed the food we'd eaten during our almost recent cruise to the Caribbean – specifically, during our ports of call in Haiti and Jamaica – and debated phoning my brothers and sisters-in-law right away… oh, and getting myself checked. After all, it was either a simple blood or breath test. Our primary care doctor preferred the blood test.

That decision was sort of a mistake. Our usual – and very good – phlebotomist was out that day having taken a sleep test (Good for her!) in a faraway part of the valley the night before and couldn't make it in, so a daily temp did the drawer. Oh! That was almost a week ago and I still have a three inch black and blue mark on the puncture site. I want my regular phlebotomist.

I know, I know, get back on topic. I didn't make those calls because my test came back negative... so it wasn't the food at the ports of call. Well, then what caused Bear's infection? WebMD tells us,

"Many people get *H. pylori* during childhood, but adults can get it, too. The germs live in the body for years before symptoms start, but most people who have it will never get ulcers."

That made sense. As a child, Bear spent his summers on his grandfather's farm and participated in whatever chores a child his age could perform. This is not to say the food or water on the farm were unclean, but

"...H. pylori bacteria may be passed from person to person through direct contact with saliva, vomit or fecal matter.... Or living with someone who has an H. pylori infection."

Thank you for that information Mayo Clinic.

Considering the existence of this type of infection wasn't discovered until 1982 and Bear was a child way before then, he may have contacted it in the manner described above.

Of course now you're wondering what the heck we were going to do about it, no matter how my poor hubby developed it since it could have drastic consequences if we didn't. (Long sentence there.) MedicineNet.com explains:

"*H. pylori* is difficult to eradicate from the stomach because it is capable of developing resistance to commonly used antibiotics. Therefore, two or more antibiotics usually are given together with a PPI and/or bismuth containing compounds to eradicate the bacterium. (Bismuth and PPIs have anti-*H. pylori* effects.)"

Is it effective? We don't know yet, since Bear is in the middle of the regiment. However, I've read that sometimes the infection can re-occur even if this treatment is successful and that the blood test is not a good choice to re-test after the medication has been finished. One step at a time, folks, one step at a time.

While I'm concerned about Bear, I also wanted to know how this might affect someone with Chronic Kidney Disease who developed it. It seems that it doesn't until you reach End Stage Chronic Kidney Disease. Since I don't know much about dialysis or any of the other end stage blood cleansing methods I can only give you information about the little I understood.

One is this conclusion from a PubMed.gov study. "The H. pylori infection rate is lower in PUD patients with CKD and ESRD than in those without CKD." Ugh! Alphabet soup. PUD is Peptic Ulcer Disease; CKD is Chronic Kidney Disease; and ESRD is End Stage Renal Disease.

But then I found a more negative study on Medscape.

"This is currently the largest nation-based study in which the risk of ESRD in *H. pylori*-infected patients was examined. *H. pylori* infection was associated with a subsequent risk of ESRD. *H. pylori*-infected patients with concomitant chronic kidney disease (CKD) or cardiovascular disease (CVD) risk factors were at higher risk of ESRD than were those who had a single CKD or CVD risk factor."

I also found it interesting that the stomach medication Omeprazole, which has just been linked to CKD, is prescribed along with antibiotics to treat H. Pylori. Now there's a Catch 22. You can take it as prescribed for your infection, the medication may damage your kidneys, or you cannot take it and have the infection damage your kidneys anyway.

2/8/16 *Still Getting Birthday Gifts... like OAB*

Bear has just spoiled me and spoiled me for this birthday. It was not a special birthday, just a birthday. His reasoning, "I'm celebrating being with you for another year." Which, of course, made me think. My first thought? I realized how much I liked being adored by the man I love.

My second? Time changes things. Your weight changes. Your hair color changes. Even your height changes. There are those that say aging is a problem. I say if you're aging, you're alive so it's not a problem, but rather something to which you need to adapt.

Part of the birthday celebration was an overnight at The Desert Rose Bed and Breakfast in Cottonwood. For a city woman like me, this was heaven. Except there were no hand rails on the steep path from the house to the rescue animals they kept on the grounds. Nor were there steps. The runoff from a recent hose cleaning of some apparatus near the house caused the loose gravel covered road to be slick. So we took teeny little 'old person' steps while the owner practically scampered. We got to see the animals, but we had to adapt how we got to them due to our age related capabilities.

The private bath was another eye opener for me. Bear opted for the room with the spa. It could have even been romantic except that there were no grab rails. We slipped, we fell, we worried if Bear broke his foot again. But it was supposed to be romantic!

Oh well. There was also the kind of shower I'd only seen in magazines. You know the kind that could easily fit six people (uh, not my style) with two separate shower heads – one on each end of the shower. This was a new toy for me, until the floor got wet. Again, no grab rails. There was no safety mat on the shower floor, either. So we tried to hold on to the walls. Hah! They were tile that was just as slippery.

You get the point? This was a beautiful, romantic, up-scale bathroom... and wasted on us because there were no safety features to accommodate our gifts from ag-ing. Of course, not everyone would have felt this way, but we each have neuropathy which can make balanc-ing difficult.

In addition to grab bars in our at home bathrooms, we have no area rugs anywhere in the house. This is to cut down on the possibility of tripping. When our primary care doctor suggested ways to prevent injuring our-selves, we listened. Bear's time flat on his back after his foot surgery convinced us we never wanted to go through that again. For me, with my 'age related' macu-lar degeneration, we also use ultra-bright LED bulbs throughout the house.

Okay, so where am I going with this? I'm circling in on the kidneys via urination. Remember the kidneys produce urine which is stored in the bladder. I wanted to know what was usual for people 'our age' and why. After all, I'd made the bathrooms as safe as possible understanding that one or the other of us was going to get up during the night to urinate.

I turned to The Cleveland Clinic for some help.

"If you're urinating more than eight times in 24 hours, that's too much. A lot depends on your age. And if you're between age 65-70 and going more than twice a night, you should make an appointment with your doctor. Also, see a doctor if you are getting up more than once a night if you are between age 60-65, and more than three times each night if you are age 70 or older. While your bladder's capacity does not necessarily decrease with age, the prevalence of overactive bladder increases with age."

Apparently, an overactive bladder may also lead to increased falls. Not fair! We're already dealing with the neuropathy to avoid this. Oh, right. "...if you're aging, you're alive so it's not a problem, but rather something to which you need to adapt."

I wonder if aging is a factor because the detrusor (bladder muscle) ages right along with the rest of you. A long time ago, I explained that my Chronic Kidney Disease was caused by nothing more than growing older. I hate to admit it, but it does make sense. All of you ages when you age, not just certain parts.

2/15/16 *The Breath of Life*

Here's hoping you had a wonderful Valentine's Day whether your Valentine was someone else or yourself. I spent years celebrating myself in various ways: an afternoon at the bookstore, an evening dancing at a new dance hall, even simply coffee with a friend I hadn't seen in a while, and enjoyed all of it.

There have been so many medical issues since last week that I wasn't quite sure which one to use as the topic of today's blog, so I decided to use the first one that came up chronologically. That was the pulmonologist. When I was in New York back in October, I experienced some shortness of breath and a burning sensation in my chest while walking at the typical New Yorker's pace (Oh, how I have forgotten what that's like.) and climbing stairs to the subway and elevated train two, three, or four times a day.

When I told the pulmonologist, who I was originally seeing for sleep apnea problems, he ordered a lung x-ray to be completed two weeks before my appointment. My lungs were perfectly clear. Yay! Hurdle number one passed.

Next, a breathing test. While I wouldn't exactly call this fascinating, it was interesting... and the technician administering it made it even more so as she explained what we were doing each step of the way and, more importantly to me, why we were doing it. I sat in a glass box while she alternately fed oxygen into my lungs or asked me to empty my lungs of the same by forcibly exhaling into a tube.

WebMd has an easy to understand explanation – the kind I like best – of these tests.

- **Nitrogen Washout:** You breathe pure oxygen, and the air you breathe out is collected and analyzed for nitrogen content.

- **Helium Dilution:** You breathe a gas mixture of helium and oxygen.

- **Body Box:** This is the most accurate of these types of tests. You sit in an enclosed chamber, made of glass or clear plastic and perform a series of small panting breaths. While very accurate, the equipment requires specially-trained technicians to operate it.

My results were not perfect, but my lung capacity was 97% which was just fine for my age. There goes that qualifier again: for my age. It's hard for me to accept that time will have an effect on your body, although it's perfectly logical. Although this is not something terrible, there have been so many borderline issues lately due to my age.

Of course you're wondering why I'm even writing about this in a Chronic Kidney Disease blog, right? To that end, I took a little jaunt into *What Is It and How Did I Get it?*

Early Stage Chronic Kidney Disease to clarify the issue for us. The first mention of the lungs was in an explanation of your nephrologist's ROS.

"Then came the Review of Systems [ROS]. My primary care physician asked me questions about my constitution, the functional habits of my body such as weight changes, fever or chills. The cardiac part of my health was covered with questions about chest pain or palpitations. Finally, the lungs were referred to with questions about coughs, shortness of breath and dyspnea."

That does still leave us with the question of why the lungs were covered at all in this examination for CKD. I found my answer in *The Book of Blogs: Moderate Stage Chronic Kidney Disease, Part 2*, in an inquiry into erythropoietin, or EPO.

"The National Kidney and Urologic Diseases Information Clearinghouse explains.

Healthy kidneys produce a hormone called erythropoietin, or EPO, which stimulates the bone marrow to produce the proper number of red blood cells needed to carry oxygen to vital organs. Diseased kidneys, however, often don't make enough EPO. As a result, the bone marrow makes fewer red blood cells."

If you have fewer red blood cells, you are carrying less oxygen to your vital organs... which are the following according to Live Science.

"The human brain….The human heart…. The job of
the kidneys is to remove waste and extra fluid from the
blood. The kidneys take urea out of the blood and com-
bine it with water and other substances to make urine.
The liver….The lungs are responsible for removing oxygen from the air we breathe and transferring it to our
blood where it can be sent to our cells. The lungs also
remove carbon dioxide, which we exhale."

Okay, so the lungs are responsible for gathering oxygen
from the air (for one thing) and healthy kidneys produce
red blood cells to carry oxygen to your vital organs
(again, for one thing). CKD reduces the oxygen you have
since it reduces your red blood cell production. Add unhealthy lungs that gather less oxygen and you're in for a
very tired time.

Keep breathing, keep enjoying, and keep on top of your
health.

2/22/16 *Will You Take a Look at That!*

Here we are again. Another Monday, another blog. Even bloggers passionate about their subjects can suffer the Monday blues, although in this case I'll bet it has to do with my CKD reduced energy level. I'd just mentioned to Bear that all I want to do is sit in the easy chair he got me last year and read the book Abby got me for Christmas while drinking coffee… well, my remaining eight ounces for the day anyway.

So I decided we'd do something a little different today. Back on March 5, 2012, I blogged about doctors being taught to be mindful. The blog was basically a New York Times article about just that.

I've noticed your comments about your doctors missing this or that which made me realize – yet again – that the usual 15 minutes allotted to each patient simply may not be enough time to really observe what's going on with you, the patient. But what could be done about that?

I was having brunch with a friend visiting from Dallas and her family when the subject arose. I wouldn't be surprised if I were the one who brought it up. But what did surprise me was that as a research assistant at the Edith O'Donnell Institute for Art History, she was involved in this program. I was flabbergasted and knew I had to share this with you.

The Art of Observation: Art Museums Partner with
Medical Schools to Teach Doctors How to Look

By Katrina Saunders

To all who have felt the healing power from a visit to
your local museum, the benefits of the art of looking
are currently being explored on a much larger scale by
museum educational departments. Partnering with
their local medical schools, art museums across the
country (and even Australia, Canada and the UK) have
developed curricula to further the observational skills of
medical students by looking at art.

The number of museums with these type of programs is
fast growing with dedicated museum staff and medical
school instructors collaborating on courses such as "Art
of Observation", which concentrates on close-looking at
works of art in museum galleries, "Art of Form", artist-
perspective led learning and making of art, and "Art of
Evaluation", round-table discussions in which students
describe their experiences.

The activity of looking is often, pardon the pun, overlooked when it comes to a medical student's jam-
packed education. Yet the benefits of training a new
generation of doctors to use their eyes means art de-
mands is beneficial to all parties involved. Through
structured viewing exercises led by expert museum
staff, medical students gain visual acumen, interpreta-
tive reasoning, and communication skills that can be

applied to patient care. Museums, in turn, can offer services that have the potential to save lives.

This type of programming began to surface in the past decade as exercises to increase visual literacy amongst medical students. Physical examination is such a large part of clinical diagnosis so medical students must learn to observe quickly, accurately and without bias. This especially becomes essential as technology and rush increasingly limit human-to-human interactions.

Dartmouth has a vibrant exchange taught between its Geisel School of Medicine and Hood Museum of Art. During "The Art of Clinical Observation" workshops, the class is divided up and museum staff host four students at a time. A cluster begins by studying one work of art for ten minutes, then each student describes it in detail to the rest of group only in terms of what is seen – without analysis or interpretation. The process repeats through the day with different works of art and ends with a discussion on how slow, careful description can be applied to diagnosing images of patients.

In 2008, Harvard published a groundbreaking study which showed that students who completed their inno-vative course "Training the Eye: Improving the Art of Physical Diagnosis" did in fact observe more than stu-dents who had not taken the course. The implications of greater observational skills all point to positive: better diagnoses leads to better patient care, extends to more efficient medical spending, and essentially makes for better doctors.

Additionally, being part of these team-building, inter-disciplinary conversations helps medical students embrace new types of thinking, ways of conversing and appreciation for different cultures. In other words, in learning to appreciate all types of art, doctors can appreciate all types of people....

Research continues to demonstrate the value of these programs, which have expanded to include a variety of topics such as empathy – how to respect and have difficult conversations with patients. Evaluative methods are still being developed that will further outline the need for medical students to slow down and hone their looking skills. The next time you visit an art museum, think of all the ways art plays a part in helping others, and be aware of how looking plays a big part of your health.

2/29/16 *Inked*

There's a woman I know, younger than I by three and a half decades, who is inked... and I mean inked. She has sleeves on both arms and (almost) a body suit. Unfortunately she's lost a job or two when narrow minded employers saw her arms, but that's not what I'm writing about today.

Oh, all right. Here are the definitions of the jargon above: inked = tattooed; sleeve= fully tattooed on the arm; body suit= tattoos on the majority of the body.

I was thinking about her the other day and that got me to thinking about tattoos and whether or not they're safe for us since we have Chronic Kidney Disease. Let's take a look at the tattooing process itself to see if there's anything there to worry about.

I turned to The Mayo Clinic for this information.

"A tattoo is a permanent mark or design made on your skin with pigments inserted through pricks into the skin's top layer. Typically, the tattoo artist uses a hand-held machine that acts much like a sewing machine, with one or more needles piercing the skin repeatedly. With every puncture, the needles insert tiny ink droplets.

The process — which is done without anesthetics — causes a small amount of bleeding and slight to potentially significant pain."

Personally, I'm too much of a scaredy cat to give tattoo-ing a try now that I know about the possibility of pain. There's enough of that in my life already... like the en-dometrial biopsy a few months ago. Ugh! But maybe you're not...

Well, why might you want a tattoo in the first place? Maybe it's an artistic requirement for your soul. Maybe it's to remind yourself of some life lesson like my New York daughter, Nima's. Or maybe it's a medical tattoo to wear rather than a medical alert bracelet.

Hmmm, I'd think again. As CKD patients, our blood is already not that pure. Remember, as I explained in *What Is It and How Did I Get It? Early Stage Chronic Kidney Disease*, "The kidneys remove these toxins (e.g. from the blood) and change them into urine ...."

Our kidneys are not functioning at the top of their game. With my current GFR of 51, my kidneys are only functioning at a teeny bit more than half capacity while still trying to filter the blood as kidneys with a GFR of 100% would. Oh, right, GFR. In *The Book of Blogs: Moderate Stage Chronic Kidney Disease, Part 1,* that's explained according to the NKDED:

"The National Kidney Disease Education Program at The U.S. Department of Health and Human Services pro-vides the following information.

A blood test checks your GFR, which tells how well your kidneys are filtering. GFR stands for glomerular filtration rate. ..."

Here's what I found on Health Impact News that makes me so leery of tattoos.

"In 2011, a study in *The British Journal of Dermatology* revealed that nanoparticles are indeed found in tattoo inks, with black pigments containing the smallest particles (white pigments had the largest particles and colored pigments were in between).

Nanoparticles are ultramicroscopic in size, making them able to readily penetrate your skin and travel to underlying blood vessels and your bloodstream. Evidence suggests that some nanoparticles may induce toxic effects in your brain and cause nerve damage, and some may also be carcinogenic."

Whenever I speak to someone who has a tattoo, they tell me the ink only goes as far as the dermis (the second layer of skin) and nowhere near the blood. I often wondered about that since the dermis is rife with blood vessels. I guess I just learned that the tattoo owners were misinformed. And why we as CKD patients should not be allowing even the possibility of more toxins entering our blood streams for our already overworked kidneys to eliminate.

Are tattoos pretty? Are they spiritual? Are they worth the risk? I found even more evidence to the contrary on WebMd.

"There are minimal side effects to laser tattoo removal. However, you should consider these factors in your decision:

The tattoo removal site is at risk for infection. You may also risk lack of complete pigment removal, and there is a slight chance that the treatment can leave you with a permanent scar...."

I'd also read on various sites that simply being tattooed may leave you open for infection if the autoclave (instrument steaming machine) or needles are not clean enough. I don't know of any sites to rate the cleanliness of tattoo parlors, but I do know infection opportunities are far more common for us as CKD patients...and they are more dangerous for us.

This paragraph from *The Book of Blogs: Moderate Stage Chronic Kidney Disease, Part 2* should clarify the why of avoiding infection possibilities.

"Think about it: your liver and your kidneys are the two most important blood filters you have. We already know we need to maintain as steady a blood pressure in the kidneys as we can to do no more damage to them. The liver does this by releasing angiotensin which constricts your blood vessels. Don't forget the liver helps maintain your blood sugars. If it can't do that due to infection, kidney function can be further reduced. The liver also filters toxins and drugs from the blood."

I wondered if I'd find enough information for a blog about CKD patients and tattoos. On the contrary, I find I could go on and on.

3/7/16 *It's National Kidney Month*

March is National Kidney Month. There's a reason there's such attention being paid to our kidneys. Last year's National Kidney Month 'Dear Abby column' explains.

"DEAR ABBY: Hypertension runs in my family, but as a pretty healthy 49-year-old, I didn't think much about it. I never realized that my pounding headaches were a direct result of high blood pressure. To make matters worse, the same high blood pressure that was causing my head to throb was also destroying my kidneys.

I wish I had known about my high blood pressure sooner and taken it seriously. When I finally learned about my kidney damage, it was too late to save them.

More than 73 million people are at risk for developing kidney disease, and I sincerely want to help them avoid this fate. My battle with kidney disease has turned me into an advocate for patients and those who are at risk. In honor of National Kidney Month in March and World Kidney Day on March 12, (Me: That was the date last year.) Will you please help me spread the word? — Lance Taylor in Minnesota

DEAR LANCE: I'm pleased to help you in this worthwhile effort. According to the National Kidney Foundation, 1 in 3 American adults is at risk for kidney disease. Major risk factors for kidney disease include diabetes, high blood pressure, a family history of kidney failure and being age 60 or older. Additional risk factors include kidney stones, smoking, obesity and cardiovascular disease.

Kidney disease often goes undetected because it lacks physical symptoms until the very late stages. By then the organs have already failed. But early detection, healthy lifestyle changes and proper treatment can slow the progress of kidney disease. Those at risk should have simple blood and urine tests to check if their kidneys are working properly.

Readers, if you are at risk, during your next physical examination, ask your health care practitioner to check your kidneys. To learn more about prevention, visit kidney.org. You will also find information about free KEEP Healthy kidney screenings in your area."

I've written about the more than 50 local offices nationwide that help the NKF provide early-detection screenings and provide other vital patient and community services. I went to the website, clicked on 'Keep Healthy Event in your area,' and up popped the locations of this particular event.

Several years ago, my daughter Nima asked if could guest blog during National Kidney Month from the perspective of someone who loves a person with CKD. These are some of the highlights of that blog.

"I have to admit when my mother first told me she had CKD I freaked out ever so slightly. My knowledge of CKD was minimal, if that, and it took more than a few times of Ma telling me that CKD was in fact manageable and not a death sentence to calm down…..

One thing I had to get used to was reminding myself to mention at doctor visits that a parent has CKD, and to please take blood work to keep an eye on my own GFR levels. Every now and then I'd also get a helpful re-minder from Ma right before a doctor visit.

I … have another resource that not everyone else has: I have a mother who is also writing a very detailed book (Working on the 4th one now.) about her experiences with discovering she had CKD. Getting a chance to read the manuscript of her upcoming book was probably where I got the meat and potatoes of my CKD educa-tion. (Nima is the professional Reader for all the CKD books I write.)

For those out there that have a loved one that was re-cently diagnosed with CKD ….don't be afraid to ask questions about what you can do to help and what you should know about how CKD affects your family mem-ber or loved one. I was always worried about tiring my mother out until she finally explained to me that as long as she gets a chance to lay down/nap before we go out, she's usually fine."

But it's not just getting tired; the following appeared on Yahoo's PRWEB on Monday, March 14, 2011. I took the online test mentioned in the article and, sure enough, I need to see an audiologist. Consider taking the online test yourself after you read this little known information about CKD patients.

"People with Chronic Kidney Disease Should Have Their Hearing Checked:

March is National Kidney Month

People with Chronic Kidney Disease (CKD) should take the Across America Hearing Check Challenge—a free, quick, and confidential online hearing test …. The non-profit Better Hearing Institute (BHI) is offering the test as part of its effort to raise awareness of the link be-tween Chronic Kidney Disease and hearing loss. March is National Kidney Month. BHI's online test will help people determine if they need a comprehensive hearing check by a hearing professional."

Every part of you is affected by your Chronic Kidney Disease. That means that everyone in your life is affect-ed by it, too. Bear knows I've got to exercise each day no matter what we have planned. My friends and family know that inviting us for dinner means I may not be able to eat what they've cooked, even if it's 'healthy.' Think about that a bit and you'll realize CKD is serious.

3/14/16   *Sex Sells...*

Well, It Keeps Us Interested Anyway

Happy Monday, blog writing day, my favorite day of the week. You know, this is the third week of National Kidney Month which brings quite a bit of kidney disease awareness activity with it. For example, this past Friday and Saturday, The National Kidney Foundation of Arizona held its 17th annual conference in partnership with The CadioRenal Society of America.

What delighted me most at the presentations was how much I understood. You see, the more I understood, the more I could bring back to you. As usual, presenter styles were varied from the one who simply read the statistics on her slideshow graphs for us to the one who told anecdotes, asked for audience participation, and had us both laughing and highly interested.

Her topic? Enhancing Intimacy and Sexuality. Her name? Robin Siegel. She is a licensed clinical social worker. Learn.org tells us, "An LCSW, or licensed clinical social worker, is a professional who provides counseling and psychosocial services to clients in clinical settings."

Ms. Siegel was actually presenting about how nephrology staff can be helpful in these areas, but quite a bit of her information was also useful for Chronic Kidney Disease patients themselves... or those that write about CKD.

Hmmm, this sounded familiar to me. Sure enough, it seems I had been thinking along the same lines when I wrote the following in *What Is It and How Did I Get It? Early Stage Chronic Kidney Disease*.

"I haven't found too much about sex that's different from the problems of non-CKD patients although with this disease there may be a lower sex drive accompanied by a loss of libido and an inability to ejaculate. Usually, these problems start with an inability to keep an erection as long as usual. The resulting impotency has a valid physical, psychological or psycho-physical cause.....

The usual remedies for E.D. can be used with CKD patients, too, but you need to make certain your urologist and your nephrologists work together, especially if your treatment involves changing medications, hormone replacement therapy or an oral medication like Viagra. ...

Women with CKD may also suffer from sexual problems, but the causes can be complicated. As with men, renal disease, diabetes and hypertension may contribute to the problem. But so can poor body image, low self-esteem, depression, stress and sexual abuse. Any chronic disease can make a man or a woman feel less sexual."

Ms. Siegel added to this by talking about possible medical intervention traumas, cultural values, and gender issues. *What Is It and How Did I Get It? Early Stage Chronic Kidney Disease* was written in 2010, although it was published in 2011. Transgender was hardly, if ever, mentioned in the news – medical or otherwise. It was the same for homosexuality. It's a different world in 2016. We talk openly about sexuality. Well, let's say many of us do. I really liked the way this presenter made it clear that these are simply part of some patients' lives and must be treated respectfully, especially when dealing specifically with their sexuality.

We agreed about intimacy, too. More from *What Is It and How Did I Get It? Early Stage Chronic Kidney Disease*:

"Sometimes people with chronic diseases can be so busy being the patient that they forget their partners have needs, too. And sometimes, remembering to stay close, really close as in hugging and snuggling, can be helpful…. The best advice I received in this area was make love even if you don't want to. Magic."

That last line is purely mine, but Ms. Siegel did talk about the snuggling and hugging from a patient point of view: allowing, giving, getting.

Something else she introduced was the different cultural values in our present day society. That's another thing that wasn't as publicly prevalent as it is today. For example, certain cultures will not permit a male doctor if the patient is female. If you belong to one of these cultures, you can simply ask for a female nephrologist in the practice or for a referral to another practice with female nephrologists if yours doesn't have any. (What??? In this day and age!!!!) According to one of my Muslim friends, there is a list of female doctors, including specialists, available in her community.

Other cultures will not allow eye contact. This is important for you to let your nephrologist know about so that he or she will not think you are avoiding topics if this is part of your culture. Sometimes written material such as handouts and pamphlets can allow you access to the same information you would have been told, too.

It seemed to me that Robin Siegel was making clear that there is no problem that can't be attended to by your nephrologist or his/her staff – even sex and intimacy – with just a bit of adapting to whatever the patient's (Oh, that means you and me.) sexuality and culture.

I have been receiving all kinds of laudatory comments about *The Book of Blogs: Moderate Stage Chronic Kidney Disease, Part 1* and *The Book of Blogs: Moderate Stage Chronic Kidney Disease, Part 2* since *SlowItDownCKD 2015* was published in digital last week. I like how that works: publish a new book and there's renewed interest in your others. Feel free to write reviews on any and all of my four CKD books.

3/21/16 *Renal Sally Port*

Sometimes things just pop into a writer's head for no reason at all. The title of this week's blog did that over and over again. Okay, I thought, I'll go with it. Only one problem: I didn't know what a sally port was and why I should be writing about a renal one.

Hmmmm, I did marry a military man. I asked. He explained but I wanted to see it in writing. Hence, this definition from The Merriam-Webster Dictionary:

1: a gate or passage in a fortified place for use by troops making a sortie

2: a secure entryway (as at a prison) that consists of a series of doors or gates

Oh, now I got it. I immediately thought of Fort Wadsworth on Staten Island where I took my little children to Civil War reenactments. There were scary, dank areas between the port and the base which were enclosed between large old gates at either end. No sun got in and it echoed in there. It was a place of fascination and fear for my little ones. What did that have to do with our kidneys?

Then I thought of having visited the friend I'd written about in the hospital when his bipolar medications needed immediate adjustment. One door was unlocked for me, I entered. That door was relocked behind me and another unlocked in front of me. That was a sally port, too.

Our gaggle of grown children has told us enough about 'Orange is the New Black' that our interest was piqued. Then Bear read my Hunter College Alumni News Letter and saw that Dascha Polanco – a major character in the series – also graduated from Hunter, although not exactly the same year I did. Those seemed like good enough reasons to give the series a try. It was set in a prison with a series of sally ports to enter or exit.

Now it was more than clear. A sally port is a security feature to guard entry and exit. Good, one half of the renal sally port secret revealed. Now, do our kidneys have sally ports?

There are three ways in or out of the kidney: the veins, the arteries, and the ureters. Let's take a look at each to see which, if any, is a sally port.

In *What Is It and How Did I Get It? Early Stage Chronic Kidney Disease*, it was explained that the renal (kidney) artery brings the unfiltered blood into the kidney:

"Your kidneys have about a million nephrons, which are those tiny structures that produce urine as part of the body's waste removal process. Each of them has a glomerulus or network of capillaries. This is where the blood from the renal artery is filtered. The glomerulus is connected to a renal tubule, something so small that it is microscopic. The renal tubule is attached to a collection area. The blood is filtered. Then the waste goes through the tubules to have water and chemicals balanced according to the body's present needs. Finally, the waste is voided via your urine to the tune of 50 gallons of fluid filtered by the kidneys DAILY. The renal vein uses blood vessels to take most of the blood back into the body."

Well, what about the renal vein? Here's how I explained it in *The Book of Blogs: Moderate Stage Chronic Kidney Disease, Part 2*:

"If you look at a picture of your kidney, you'll see that blood with wastes in it is brought to the kidneys by the renal artery and clean blood is exited from the kidneys by the renal vein. Your kidneys are already compromised which means they are not doing such a great job of filtering your blood."

Well, if the renal artery is the sally port for the blood entering your kidneys, the renal vein sounds like the more important renal sally port since it's allowing that poorly filtered blood back into your blood stream.

Oh wait, we forgot the ureter. There's an explanation from *SlowItDownCKD 2015* about that.

Many thanks to the ever reliable MedicineNet for the following.

"A hollow organ in the lower abdomen that stores urine. The kidneys filter waste from the blood and produce urine, which enters the bladder through two tubes, called ureters. Urine leaves the bladder through another tube, the urethra. In women, the urethra is a short tube that opens just in front of the vagina. In men, it is longer, passing through the prostate gland and then the penis. Also known as urinary bladder and vesical."

Uh, no, there's nothing in that description that indicates the urethra is a sally port.

So... the renal vein then. How does this poor excuse for allowing filtered blood back into our blood stream affect us? (I do admit that it seems it's more the fault of the damaged glomeruli than the renal vein acting as a sally port.)

For one thing, we become one of the one-in-three at risk for Chronic Kidney Disease ... and that's only in America. For another, our bodily functions differently as do our minds. I included this not-so-pleasing information from EurekAlert! in a 2012 post in *The Book of Blogs: Moderate Stage Chronic Kidney Disease, Part 1:*

"Decreased kidney function leads to

decreased cognitive functioning

Decreased kidney function is associated with decreased cognitive functioning in areas such as global cognitive ability, abstract reasoning and verbal memory, according to a study led by Temple University. This is the first study describing change in multiple domains of cognitive functioning in order to determine which specific abilities are most affected in individuals with impaired renal function."

But there's more. According to the National Kidney Foundation, this is what is our kidneys are NOT doing for us as well as they should since we have CKD:

- Regulate the body's fluid levels

- Filter wastes and toxins from the blood

- Release a hormone that regulates blood pressure

- Activate Vitamin D to maintain healthy bones

- Release the hormone that directs production of red blood cells

- Keep blood minerals in balance (sodium, phosphorus, potassium)

I'm glad I got the term renal sally port out of my system, but I wish the news had been better.

3/28/16 *How Sweet It Was*

I've had an interesting turn around in my health this last week of National Kidney Month. You did know it's still National Kidney Month, right? You did go get yourself tested for Chronic Kidney Disease, didn't you? Hurry up! There're only four more days left to National Kidney Month. You know I'm joking about this month being *the* time to get yourself tested, but I'm serious (unfortunately, sometimes dead serious) about getting yourself tested.

I know, I know, I'm preaching to the choir. But how many of you have told your friends, neighbors, family, and co-workers about just how simple – and important – these tests are. Let's not let them become one of the 31 million with Chronic Kidney Disease or worse, one of those that don't know they have it.

Excuse me while I step off my soap opera. Now, where was I? Oh, yes, the – ahem – interesting turn around in my health this month.

Okay, this is twofold. The first part is the weight. You think I've been having trouble keeping that in check since I started blogging four years ago, don't you? I mean because I write about it so much. The truth is it's been much, much longer than that. Even way back in college when I was a size 7 for one day, I weighed more than 'the charts' said I should by 20 pounds or so. I looked good, I felt good, and my mom kept telling me I had 'heavy bones,' so I let it go. Who knew any better back then?

What's so bad about the extra weight you ask? You do know obesity is one of the causes of CKD, don't you? Don't feel bad if you didn't. I didn't. I just started noticing it showing up in the research in the last couple of years. That doesn't mean it wasn't there. It just means I never saw it if it was.

I mentioned weight in passing a few times in *What Is It and How Did I Get It? Early Stage Chronic Kidney Disease*. This is from my first nephrologist's report:

"The report, of course, ended with a one – two punch: I would need to exercise for at least 30 minutes a day and possibly decrease food portions, so I could lose weight (all right already! I got it!) for better blood pressure and renal function."

Better blood pressure and renal function? That's when my battle with the numbers became real. And that's when weighing and measuring food according to the renal diet allotments worked for a while... until I thought I could eye measure. So I went back to weighing and measuring... and it worked...until bomb shell number two fell in my lap: pre-diabetes.

In *The Book of Blogs: Moderate Chronic Kidney Disease, Part 1*, The National Institutes of Health helped me explain why this combination of excess weight and pre-diabetes was a problem for CKD patients:

"High blood glucose and high blood pressure damage the kidneys' filters. When the kidneys are damaged, proteins leak out of the kidneys into the urine. The urinary albumin test detects this loss of protein in the urine. Damaged kidneys do not do a good job of filtering out wastes and extra fluid. Wastes and fluid build up in your blood instead of leaving the body in urine."

Let's backtrack just a bit here. What does high blood glucose have to do with this? Well, that's what is tested to measure your A1C, which determines whether or not you have diabetes... or even pre-diabetes.

Back to *The Book of Blogs: Moderate Chronic Kidney Disease, Part 2.* This time for me to decry my A1C woes:

"This time I went to WebMD for a simple explanation. In addition to learning that pre diabetes means your glucose, while not diabetic, is higher than normal, I found this interesting statement.

'When glucose builds up in the blood, it can damage the tiny blood vessels in the kidneys, heart, eyes, and nervous system.'"

What I learned from my primary care physician on my last visit is that the A1C is not the only measure of diabetes. Although my blood glucose readings are still in the pre-diabetes range according to the A1C, my daily readings have sometimes gone over the 126 that's considered diabetes. My head is spinning here. No one ever mentioned that magic number to me before.

I decided to conduct a little experiment last night. We know that high blood glucose is the result of sugar, but did you know that most carbohydrates turn into sugar? Last night I ate a chocolate bar and devoured at least half a dozen Saltines. This morning, when I pricked my finger and tested the blood, the reading was 129. Damn! Someone had to be the guinea pig and I volunteered myself… but all I'd proven was that sugar and carbs raise your blood sugar pretty quickly.

Now here's the kicker. This is from *SlowItDownCKD 2015*:

"The Brits do a masterful job of explaining this effectively. The following is from *Patient*.

'A raised blood sugar (glucose) level that occurs in people with diabetes can cause a rise in the level of some chemicals within the kidney. These chemicals tend to make the glomeruli (Me here inserting my two cents: what filters the blood in your kidneys) more 'leaky' which then allows albumin to leak into the urine. In addition, the raised blood glucose level may cause some proteins in the glomeruli to link together. These 'cross-linked' proteins can trigger a localised scarring process. This scarring process in the glomeruli is called glomerulosclerosis. It usually takes several years for glomerulosclerosis to develop and it only happens in some people with diabetes.'"

My nephrologist told me to cut out sugar and carbs to lose weight. I'd already cut out sugar, so I cut out (or at least drastically down on) carbs. The result: a very slow weight loss. Of course, this is new to me so I don't know if that two pound weight loss in a month will continue every month, but I'm willing to give it a try. Say, that'll have a possible effect on eliminating the diabetes, too!

4/4/16 *If Only It Had Been an April Fool's Joke*

I thought it was a mean April Fool's joke, but it wasn't. I thought I'd heard wrong, but I hadn't. I thought this was a mistake, but it wasn't. Both of my brothers have Parkinson's disease. Now another non-blood family member had just been diagnosed with the same disease... out of the blue, unexpectedly, seemingly impossibly.

PD – Parkinson's disease in this case, not to be confused with Peritoneal Dialysis – is not only a genetic driven disease, but sometimes an environmentally driven one. This relative had been in Viet Nam. This relative had had the job of patrolling the areas of the jungle that had been saturated with Agent Orange to defoliate for better visibility. He'd done that every 15 days for over a year. 45 years later, he's been diagnosed with PD. A coincidence? Not according to his neurologist who immediately told him to file disability papers with the Veterans' Administration based on this information.

My mind was tripping over itself trying to explain this all to you – and to me. I needed to know just what this Agent Orange was. Dictionary.com explained:

"a powerful herbicide and defoliant containing trace amounts of dioxin, a toxic impurity suspected of causing serious health problems, including cancer and genetic damage, in some persons exposed to it and birth defects in their offspring: used by U.S. armed forces during the Vietnam War to defoliate jungles."

Dioxin? What's that? It sounded familiar, but I couldn't quite remember. I wanted a definition I could understand so I jumped right over to MedicineNet.

"One of a number of poisonous petroleum-derived chemicals which are produced when herbicides (substances used for killing plants) are made or when plastics are burned. Dioxins are chemically dibenzo-p-dioxins...."

Poisonous. That made me wonder what this poison could do to a human body. This is the list of those possibilities I found on the Veterans' Administration's Agent Orange website:

AL Amyloidosis, A rare disease caused when an abnormal protein, amyloid, enters tissues or organs

Chronic B-cell Leukemias, A type of cancer which affects white blood cells

Chloracne (or similar acneform disease), A skin condition that occurs soon after exposure to chemicals and looks like common forms of acne seen in teenagers.

Diabetes Mellitus Type 2 (Me here: Diabetes is the number one cause of CKD.), A disease characterized by high blood sugar levels resulting from the body's inability to respond properly to the hormone insulin

Hodgkin's Disease, A malignant lymphoma (cancer) characterized by progressive enlargement of the lymph nodes, liver, and spleen, and by progressive anemia

Ischemic Heart Disease, A disease characterized by a reduced supply of blood to the heart, that leads to chest pain

Multiple Myeloma, A cancer of plasma cells, a type of white blood cell in bone marrow

Non-Hodgkin's Lymphoma, A group of cancers that affect the lymph glands and other lymphatic tissue

Parkinson's disease (My bolding), **A progressive disorder of the nervous system that affects muscle movement**

Peripheral Neuropathy, Early-Onset, A nervous system condition that causes numbness, tingling, and motor weakness.

Porphyria Cutanea Tarda, A disorder characterized by liver dysfunction and by thinning and blistering of the skin in sun-exposed areas.

Prostate Cancer, Cancer of the prostate; one of the most common cancers among men

Respiratory Cancers (includes lung cancer), Cancers of the lung, larynx, trachea, and bronchus

Soft Tissue Sarcomas (other than osteosarcoma, chondrosarcoma, Kaposi's sarcoma, or mesothelioma), A group of different types of cancers in body tissues such as muscle, fat, blood and lymph vessels, and connective tissues

My heart sank. But what of the Parkinson's patient who also has Chronic Kidney Disease. How will the CKD be affected by the PD? We already know we, as CKD patients, can develop muscle weakness and tiredness due to our poorly filtered blood (We know you're trying, damaged kidneys.). Parkinson's does the same. I couldn't even image being the victim of doubly weak muscles.

I found a number of scholarly studies on the effects of PD on those with CKD, but each site was of the purchase-the-study-if-you-want-to-read-it type. That was a bit too costly for me. I still needed more information though.

From the National Institutes of Health, I discovered that renal disease does contribute to "excessive daytime sleepiness in PD patients," although I was actually looking for PD effects on CKD. We're already tired. Does this mean we'll be even more tired should we develop PD?

Ready to be shocked? Here we go: "ESRD is significantly associated with an increased risk of Parkinson's disease. Close surveillance for Parkinson's disease should be considered for patients with ESRD." Oh great. As if we didn't have enough to worry about. By the way, ESRD is end stage renal disease. Once again, the National Institutes of Health gave us this information.

While not exactly on topic, I found this disturbing similarity between the two diseases:

"Frustratingly, for kidney failure patients, the routine laboratory tests are almost never abnormal, and only hint abnormality when the failure process has already begun. In Parkinson's disease, as in kidney failure, a 'threshold' of cells must be lost before one manifests symptoms."

There's more, much more, from The Center for Movement Disorder and Neurorestoration.

Now I'm beginning to wonder if the drugs for Parkinson's exit the body through the kidneys, but I think that's a topic for another blog. I also realize that having CKD may affect PD more than PD may affect CKD. Sometimes, I surprise myself with what I learn.

4/11/16 *All Is Not Lost*

Last week, I told you the bad news about yet another member of my family being stricken with Parkinson's disease.

I didn't know much about the medication to ameliorate the symptoms of the disease, so that's what I'm exploring this week. But… we need to go back a little bit to see what this myriad of symptoms consists of. Let's start with a simple definition of Parkinson's disease. We'll call it PD, but remember that doesn't mean peritoneal dialysis in this particular blog.

According to Consumer Health Digest,

"Parkinson's disease is a disorder of the nervous system that progresses with time. It primarily affects the movement of a person. It develops steadily typically beginning with a slight tremor in one hand. Aside from causing tremor that is the most well-known sign of the disease, it also usually causes stiffness or the slowing of movement. During the early stages, the face may show very little, or no expression at all and the arms may not swing when the affected individual walks. Speech can also become softer or slurred."

I do see most of these symptoms in the newly diagnosed member of my family. (Anecdote to lighten this heavy blog: one of my brothers has the 'no expression' symptom. A young fellow snidely called him stone face. I quietly told him my brother has Parkinson's and can't smile. My brother laughed. I laughed. Finally, the young fellow laughed, too.) What else?

The Mayo Clinic answered my question:

"Tremor. A tremor, or shaking, usually begins in a limb, often your hand or fingers. You may notice a back-and-forth rubbing of your thumb and forefinger, known as a pill-rolling tremor. One characteristic of Parkinson's disease is a tremor of your hand when it is relaxed (at rest).

Slowed movement (bradykinesia). Over time, Parkinson's disease may reduce your ability to move and slow your movement, making simple tasks difficult and time-consuming. Your steps may become shorter when you walk, or you may find it difficult to get out of a chair. Also, you may drag your feet as you try to walk, making it difficult to move.

Rigid muscles. Muscle stiffness may occur in any part of your body. The stiff muscles can limit your range of motion and cause you pain.

Impaired posture and balance. Your posture may become stooped, or you may have balance problems as a result of Parkinson's disease.

Loss of automatic movements. In Parkinson's disease, you may have a decreased ability to perform unconscious movements, including blinking, smiling or swinging your arms when you walk.

Speech changes. You may have speech problems as a result of Parkinson's disease. You may speak softly, quickly, slur or hesitate before talking. Your speech may be more of a monotone rather than with the usual inflections.

Writing changes. It may become hard to write, and your writing may appear small."

Oh, I'd seen all of these in him. Maybe he should have taken his neurologist's suggestion that he begin medication, but it hadn't been explained very well. Actually, it hadn't been explained at all. So what was it?

Oh, my, there are so many different medications listed depending upon your unique set of symptoms. The most common is a combination of L-dopa and carbidopa according to WebMD.

"Levodopa (also called L-dopa) is the most commonly prescribed and most effective drug for controlling the symptoms of Parkinson's disease, particularly bradykinesia and rigidity.

Levodopa is transported to the nerve cells in the brain that produce dopamine. It is then converted into dopamine for the nerve cells to use as a neurotransmitter.

...carbidopa increases its effectiveness and prevents or lessens many of the side effects of levodopa, such as nausea, vomiting, and occasional heart rhythm disturbances."

Hey, wait a minute! Drugs.com is emphatic that you tell your doctor if you have diabetes or kidney disease BEFORE this is prescribed for you. Ummmmm, we have CKD; that's kidney disease... and many of us have diabetes which caused the CKD. There's the same warning about kidney disease on the same site for carbidopa.

Last week, I discovered that if you have ESRD, you'll more likely to develop Parkinson's. This brings up more and more questions for me. My newly diagnosed with Parkinson's family member doesn't have CKD, but I do... and you do. What if we reach end stage? What if we develop Parkinson's? You know what? That's what the specialists are for.

Looking at the medical treatments of a disease that's fairly new to me, what I've realized is that your drug treatment has to be specifically tailored for you. You may have symptoms my loved one doesn't; he may have symptoms you don't. You may well tolerate a drug; he may need secondary drugs to counteract the side effects of the same drug. He may well tolerate a drug you just can't without several secondary drugs to counteract the side effects.

When one of my brothers told me this is a complicated disease, I don't think I realized just how complicated.

I'm not a doctor as I keep repeating. I know when we need one, a specialist at that, and now is the time.

Does that mean lose hope? Of course not, drugs are only one type of treatment for Parkinson's. There's a whole new field of physical therapy especially for movement disorders. Most of these will cover:

Strengthening

Flexibility

Balance

Gait Training

Transfer Training

I've been watching my loved one struggle to lift himself off the couch, navigate turns while walking, and keep his balance. It could be heart breaking if we didn't know help is available. The program he'll be attending is intensive, four weeks of four days a week. The retired teacher over here told him to think of it as school.

4/18/16 *Why Not Here?*

Having had no particular medical issue of my own this week – finally! – and none for anyone else in the family, I was casting about for something I'd like to write about when I found this in my files. It's from SBS, which is self-described as, "...multilingual and multicultural radio and television services that inform, educate and entertain all Australians and, in doing so, reflect Australia's multicultural society."

"'The State of the Nation: Chronic Kidney Disease in Australia' report by Kidney Health Australia shows while one in 10 adults have kidney disease, only one in 100 know they have it. But Kidney Health Australia medical director Tim Mathews said that could be about to change thanks to a new take-home test distributed by pharmacists.

'Pharmacists have an opportunity to identify people at high risk of kidney trouble – those who present with a prescription for diabetes and for high blood pressure are the two groups we're focusing on,' Dr Mathews said. 'So that's an opportunity for them to have a dialogue with the patient and see if they've had their kidneys checked, and if not, offer them a urine test which the patient then buys and takes home to test in their own privacy. At the moment we know in General Practice, only 40 per cent of diabetics are having a urine test each year – we would hope to push that number up by this program. '"

Of course, I know that we're not in Australia and that this is from almost two years ago, but think of it! Here we are desperate to spread Chronic Kidney Awareness so that people will know to be checked for the disease while the Australians are already doing something about people getting tested.

Why can't we do that? Or are we already doing that? If we aren't, why not? It just seemed such a simple aid to informing people they need to be tested.

I've written four books about CKD and I know I haven't covered this possibility in *What Is It and How Did I Get It? Early Stage Chronic Kidney Disease*, *The Book of Blogs: Moderate Stage Chronic Kidney Disease, Parts 1* and *2*, or *SlowItDownCKD 2015*. Why not? Because the idea is just so simple, so obvious, that I never thought of it. Let's see if anyone else in the U.S. has.

Hmmm, I did find this from EurekAlert:

"Pharmacists who screened at-risk patients for chronic kidney disease (CKD) found previously unrecognized disease in 1 of every 6.4 patients tested, according to a study to be published in the January/February 2016 issue of the *Canadian Pharmacists Journal*."

Sorry, wrong country – although we're at least on the right continent now. I think I just found one... nope, that's in England. Wait, there's something in the *American Journal of Kidney Disease*... oh, it's an editorial proposing pharmacists keep on the lookout for those at risk for CKD. Will you look at that! This was proposed in 2004, a dozen years ago. Canada, UK, Canada. No, nothing for the USA.

I know my pharmacist is very, very careful to check that the drugs I'm prescribed are those that will not harm my kidneys. You've probably already read several of my blogs about that. In the last one, I wrote about how a doctor covering for my primary care physician would not listen when I told him I had CKD and that my pharmacist told me point blank not to buy the drug he prescribed, then called him to make certain he understood why this drug was not one for CKD patients. He didn't listen to me; she did... and then made him listen to her.

I'm lucky. I have never felt alone, not even with the CKD diagnose. But some of my readers have let me know how very alone they feel with their illness even though family and friends are supportive. That's why I want to let you know about The National Kidney Foundation's Peers. The following is from their website.

"Do you need help adjusting to life with kidney disease? Or want to learn more about treatment options? NKF Peers is a FREE, telephone-based peer support program from the National Kidney Foundation. The program matches those in need of support with a peer mentor who has been through a similar situation. You'll connect with your mentor through a free, private phone system so you won't have to disclose your personal phone number....

About NKF Peers

- A national, telephone-based peer support program from the National Kidney Foundation

- Connects people who want support with someone who has been there

- Helps people adjust to living with chronic kidney disease, kidney failure, or a kidney transplant.

Also offers support to those considering living kidney donation or who have been have been living kidney donors.

How do participants interact with each other?

- Participants are connected through a toll-free, automated telephone system. No one discloses personal phone numbers or incurs long-distance charges.

- The automated telephone system allows participants to leave voicemail messages for their partners and block calls at certain hours.

- Telephone services are provided free-of-charge by the NKF.

To learn more: Call 855-653-7337 (855-NKF-PEER) or email nkfpeers@kidney.org"

Of course, you can always drop a question or a comment on *SlowItDownCKD*'s Facebook page and I'll research whatever you're asking about... with the provision that you understand I am not a doctor and that you need to speak with your nephrologist before taking any action on my advice. If it's private, you can email me at *SlowItDownCKD@gmail.com* ...with the same provision. By the way, I'm available 24 hours a day, seven days a week.

4/25/16 *Rain, Rain, Go Away...*

We had a day of rain. I know that's not a terribly unusual statement, but this is Arizona. July and August are our rainy months; it's only April. Well, we do know the climate is changing. .. and we do know it's affecting our health. That includes the rain. How? Most often – aside from sun showers – if it's raining, the sun isn't shining.

So? What's the big deal, I can almost hear you ask. You're not out there getting your 10 to 15 sunscreen-less-before-the-day-heats-up minutes of the best source of vitamin D if it's raining, my friends. Of course, there are supplements and loads of us, like me, take them. But the gold standard? Natural sunlight.

Bear even got me a hammock chair so I could sit in the sun really, really comfortably for my 10 to 15 minutes. So comfortably, that I found him in my chair once too often when I wanted to be in it and bought him one of his own. Now we can get at least 10 to 15 minutes together each day.

According to the National Kidney Foundation:

"Researchers found that those who were deficient in vitamin D were more than twice as likely to develop albuminuria (a type of protein in the urine) over a period of five years. Albuminuria is an early indication of kidney damage as healthy kidneys capture protein for use in the body.

'There have been a number of studies establishing a relationship between vitamin D levels and kidney disease,' said Thomas Manley, Director of Scientific Activities for the National Kidney Foundation. 'This study supports that relationship and shows that a low vitamin D level increases the likelihood of developing protein in the urine, even among a general population.'"

That's not all, folks. I jumped back to my very first Chronic Kidney Disease book, *What Is It and How Did I Get It? Early Stage Chronic Kidney Disease* for more information about vitamin D and our kidneys:

"The kidneys produce calcitrol which is the active form of vitamin D. The kidneys are the organs that transfer this vitamin from your food and skin [sunshine provides it to your skin] into something your body can use. Both vitamin D and calcium are needed for strong bones. It is yet another job of your kidneys to keep your bones strong and healthy. Should you have a deficit of Vitamin D, you'll need to be treated for this, in addition for any abnormal level of calcium or phosphates. The three work together. Vitamin D enables the calcium from the food you eat to be absorbed in the body. CKD may leech the calcium from your bones and body. Phosphate levels can rise since this is stored in the blood and the bones as is calcium. With CKD, it's hard to keep the phosphate levels normal, so you may develop itchiness since the concentration of urea builds up and begins to crystallize through the skin. This is called pruritus."

All for the lack of a little sunshine! Yes, I am being dramatic and, yes, you can take supplements, but that's like drinking juice instead of eating the whole fruit and expecting the same benefits.

In *The Book of Blogs: Moderate Stage Chronic Kidney Disease, Part 2*, I wrote the following:

"I have many more articles in front of me, so I'm going to simply list the areas in which low vitamin D is involved.

- cardiovascular

- Chronic Kidney Disease {The purpose of this blog, lest we forget}

- health hip fracture risk

- hepatitis B {Have you decided to take the inoculation against this?}

- hypertension

- stroke

Got how dangerous low levels of vitamin D can be? Good."

Uh-huh, vitamin D is a big deal... especially for us since we have CKD. According to the National Institutes of Health,

"A growing body of research suggests that vitamin D might play some role in the prevention and treatment of type 1 … and type 2 diabetes …, hypertension …, glucose intolerance…, multiple sclerosis …, and other medical conditions…."

Oh, there's also a good possibility that vitamin D deficiency is a factor in obesity. As one who is constantly attempting to lose weight, I have one thing to say about that, "Go.sit.in.the.sun."

I've been getting questions about transplantation, as in how to, what it entails, and who to contact. I don't have the answers, but the Erma Bombeck Project does. This is from an email I received from The National Kidney Foundation of Arizona:

"Today, over 100,000 Americans are waiting for a life-saving kidney transplant. The Erma Bombeck Project provides facts and reliable resources to help individuals save a life – whether by registering to be a non-living organ donor, or considering the gift of life through living donation. The project aims to narrow the gap between the number of individuals desperately waiting for a kidney and the number of kidneys available.

We invite you to visit the new, improved site www.ErmaBombeckProject.org where you can find features like:

Facts on kidney donation
A free, downloadable Living Donor Guide

Living Donor Educational Videos
Links to additional resources"

I urge you to take a look at the site should this interest you ... and I really hope it interests you.

In a few days, I'll be on my way to San Antonio – specifically Lackland Air Force Base – where my step daughter's sweetheart will graduate from basic training. I'm eager to try out my on-the-road exercise and food ideas during the 14 plus hour drive. Bear is going too, of course, so I'll have my staunchest supporter with me. And Lara is very respectful of my needs and has even offered to water walk with me since the hotel has a pool. This should be fun! Anyone have any sightseeing recommendations?

5/2/16 *Maybe This One?*

Hi y'all! I'm still deep in the heart of Texas and will tell
you about it next week. My friend Beth, a fellow Land-
mark graduate and the originator of the Facebook
page *Morning Gratitude*, offers a product I am eager to
explore this week. She is excited about its health and
weight loss benefits. This seems to be the national pas-
time these days, but I must say each person I've spoken
with is delighted with the results of their products... but
they don't have Chronic Kidney Disease.

You might remember that last November I spent the
month writing about different products. They sounded
good, healthy, and I wondered if I could use them. The
answer? No, no, no, and no. They were either way out
of the guidelines for phosphorous, protein, potassium,
and/or sodium on my renal diet or they were out of
guidelines for the pre-diabetic diet I've incorporated
with my renal diet. That incorporation took me over a
year to figure out so there was no way I was going to
violate it. I have been having some success slowly losing
weight and bringing my blood sugar in line by cutting
out sugar and most complex starches, as well as contin-
uing to exercise. (Yes, that's a not at all veiled hint.)

Beth, a friend for three years, is so happy with her
brand – Plexus Worldwide – that she's become a dis-
tributor. Similar to some of the other brands I explored
for CKD patients in *SlowItDownCKD 2015*, Plexus
Worldwide offers many different products. I took an in-

depth look at the one that seemed to be the basic product: Plexus 96.

According to Beth's Plexus website, this particular product contains alpha lipoic acid, chlorogenic acid, garcina cambogia, whey protein, green lipped mussel, aloe vera, and grape seed extract. Stop. What is chlorogenic acid? Anyone? No one knows? Let's find out together then.

This ingredient is a miracle according to the internet. It supposedly helps you lose weight, is an antioxidant, cleanses the liver... shall I go on? I liked almost everything I read about it except that it is not yet approved by the Food and Drug Administration. I never used to care about that. Now I have CKD, so I do. Why? If a supplement is not approved, there's no way to know how to adjust the dosage for your (and my) poorly performing kidneys.

In addition, the UK Medicines Information (UKMI) for pharmacists NHS healthcare professionals published the following finding on April 8, 2013:

"Limited laboratory studies appear to suggest that chlorogenic acid can cause liver or kidney changes. Until more is known, it would be prudent to avoid GCE in patients with pre-existing liver or kidney disease."

*GCE is Green Coffee Extract, the source of chlorogenic acid.

Right out of the gate, this is not a product for people with CKD. I would go on, but I think it might be better to explore another of Plexus's products. You know what they say, 'One bad apple doesn't spoil the bunch.'

I liked the sound of the Plexus Slim. When I looked at the ingredient list, the first thing I saw was chlorogenic acid. We know we can't have this, but let's look at one more ingredient just for the heck of it. Here's one I often hear about: garcinia cambogia. I went directly to their website at to look for possible side effects. Uh-oh:

"Increases risk for rhabdomyolysis, a skeletal muscle disease that causes the muscles to release proteins into the bloodstream leading to kidney malfunction."

Ladies and gentlemen, our protein intake is restricted because we have CKD. Why would we take a chance on increasing the protein in our bodies? Here's a reminder from *What Is It and How Did I Get It? Early Stage Chronic Kidney Disease* about why we need to limit our protein.

"So, why is protein limited? One reason is that it is the source of a great deal of phosphorus. Another is that a number of nephrons were already destroyed before you were even diagnosed. Logically, those that remain compensate for those that are no longer viable. The remaining nephrons are doing more work than they were meant to. Just like a car that is pushed too hard, there will be constant deterioration if you don't stop pushing.

The idea is to stop pushing your remaining nephrons to work even harder in an attempt to slow down the advancement of your CKD. Restricting protein is a way to reduce the nephrons' work."

Beth did tell me she didn't know if Plexus would be good for Chronic Kidney Disease patients. Okay, we'll look at just one more product before we call it a day. The name drew me to the product and the ingredient silica turned me away again. I'm referring to Plexus X Factor which is described on the website in the following manner.

"Plexus X Factor is a turbocharged multivitamin and antioxidant supplement with a never-before-seen formulation of a patented aloe blend and New Zealand Blackcurrant of which results in vastly improved absorption and assimilation for optimal nutrition and wellness protection."

Wait a minute. I remember having read something about silica. It wasn't complimentary. Found it! It was listed under Side Effects and Precautions of Silica Supplements along with a warning that this is not FDA approved.

"Kidney Function. Some medical teams have also expressed concerns that using silica supplements for a prolonged period of time may cause severe kidney trouble. People who take these supplements have reported kidney stones and medical professionals believe it may be because of a buildup of extra silica within the body as only small quantities are required for proper bodily functions. General kidney deterioration can also occur over time if there is excess silica in the body and this condition is irreversible."

Are you getting the feeling that none of these new products for health improvement and/or weight are acceptable for CKD patients? I am and it has to do with the unregulated herbs that may cause or worsen kidney damage. What do you say we quit while we're ahead? Of course, those without CKD need to decide for themselves if this is something they'd like to try.

5/9/16 *Deep in the Heart of Texas*

Last week I wrote that I'd tell you about our Texas trip this week and that's just what I'll do... sort of. We were in San Antonio for the Air Force Basic Training Graduation of a close family friend. I hadn't wanted to go. The rest of the family was driving 14 hours straight. I thought they were insane.

It turned out I was right about that, but I am glad I went anyway. The next day, our friend proposed to his girl-friend – who just happened to be our daughter – at The Riverwalk's Secret Waterfall, Airmen escort and all. THAT was worth the ride. And we got to know his family better, understand them more, and value their compa-ny. As they say in the ad, "Priceless."

There was only one fly in the ointment. While the tem-perature was manageable for us since we live in Arizo-na, the humidity was not for the same reason. For my other than U.S. readers (and there are quite a few of them since I have 107,000 readers in 106 countries), Arizona's usual humidity is low, very low. We do have a three minute rainy season in August (Okay, maybe it's a teensy bit more than three minutes.) when it rises, but that's not the norm.

Last week, the humidity in San Antonio, Texas, was be-tween 68% and 72%. Even the air conditioning in the hotel bowed before it. Our Airman had scheduled the entire weekend for us: The Airman's run on an open field, late lunch at a restaurant with no available indoor seating, graduation on the parade field, an afternoon on The Riverwalk. There's more, but you get the idea. All of it outdoors, all of it in 68% to 72% humidity, all of it uncomfortable as can be.

And, it turns out, all of it not great for a Chronic Kidney Disease patient. Why? Well, that's the topic of today's blog. ResearchGate published a study from the *Asian Journal of Pharmaceutical and Clinical Research* from February of 2014 (That's over two years ago, friends.) which included the following in the conclusion:

"Our data suggest that burden of renal diseases may increase as period of hot weather becomes more frequent. This is further aggravated if age advanced and people with chronic diseases like diabetes and hypertension."

That makes sense, but *how* will this happen exactly? I included this June, 2010, article in *The Book of Blogs: Moderate Chronic Kidney Disease, Part 1*. Apparently, heat (and humidity) has been an acknowledged threat to our kidneys for longer than we'd thought.

"....Dr. HL Trivedi of the Institute of Kidney Diseases and Research Centre (IKDRC) said, '.... Rapid water loss causes the kidney's functioning to slow down, resulting in temporary or permanent kidney failure.'

Extreme heat causes rapid water loss, resulting in acute electrolyte imbalance. The kidney, unable to cope with the water loss, fails to flush out the requisite amount of Creatinine and other toxins from the body. Coupled with a lack of consistent water intake, this brings about permanent or temporary kidney failure, explain experts."

The article is from "Daily News & Analysis."

By the time *The Book of Blogs: Moderate Chronic Kidney Disease, Part 2* was ready for publication, the (then) spokesman for The National Kidney Foundation – Dr. Leslie Spry – had this to say about heat and humidity:

"Heat illness occurs when body temperature exceeds a person's ability to dissipate that heat and is commonly diagnosed when the body temperature approaches 104 degrees Fahrenheit and when humidity is greater than 70 percent. Once the humidity is that high, sweating becomes less effective at dispersing body heat, and the core body temperature begins to rise."

Oh, so humidity affects sweating and body heat rises. Humidity greater than 70%. That covers almost the entire time we were in Texas. Well, what's the connection between heat illness and CKD then?

The CDC offers the following advice to avoid heat illness:

"People with a chronic medical condition are less likely to sense and respond to changes in temperature. Also, they may be taking medications that can worsen the impact of extreme heat. People in this category need the following information.

- Drink more water than usual and don't wait until you're thirsty to drink.

- Check on a friend or neighbor, and have someone do the same for you.

- Check the local news for health and safety updates regularly.

- Don't use the stove or oven to cook——it will make you and your house hotter.

- Wear loose, lightweight, light-colored clothing.

- Take cool showers or baths to cool down.

- Seek medical care immediately if you or someone you know experiences symptoms of heat-related illness

Uh-oh, we're already in trouble. Look at the first suggestion: our fluid intake is restricted to 64 oz. (Mine is, check with your nephrologist for yours.) I know I carefully space out my fluids – which include anything that can melt to a liquid – to cover my entire day. I can't drink more water than usual and, sometimes – on those rare occasions when I've been careless – have to wait until I'm thirsty to drink.

Diabetes is the foremost cause of CKD. I was curious how heat affected blood sugar so I popped over to Information about Diabetes and found this:

1. If our body is low on fluids, the kidneys receive less blood flow and work less effectively. This might cause blood glucose concentrations to rise.

2. If someone's blood sugar is already running high in the heat, not only will they lose water through sweat but they might urinate more frequently too, depleting their body's fluids even more.

There's more at the website if this interests you.

So, pretty much, the way to deal with heat and humidity having an effect on your (and my) CKD is to avoid it. That doesn't mean you have to move, you know. Stay in air conditioning as long as you can so your body is not overheated and can better handle this kind of weather. Wearing a hat and cool clothes will also help. I certainly learned the value of wearing cotton this past week. It's a fabric that breathes.

5/16/16 *It's Not Lemonade*

"Why drinking water with lemon is good for you," screamed The Chicago Tribune at me today. Hmmm, I'd been wondering about that. Last week, I'd attended the 60th birthday celebration of my friend Naomi. She is studying nutritional counseling. That's right: studying at age 60. As you can tell, no grass grows under the feet of the people in my social circle.

The celebration was held in one of the beautiful resorts out here in Arizona, The Sanctuary, in The Jade Bar to be exact. It was an odd location since this bar was long and narrow with couches and comfortable chairs lined up, but no place to mingle or chat in small groups. We ended up climbing over each other just to get to the rest room. Yet, my friend came running up to greet us.

Why? She wanted to know if I was drinking the water with lemon first thing in the morning as she'd suggested when I was a test case for one of her classes. She explained to me how important it was to people and her friends Lily and Patty leaned over to verify with their own personal anecdotes.

According to Tribune's article,

"'Health experts say the acidity of the lemons improves digestion. Lemons contain potent antioxidants, which can also protect against disease,' says Dr. Jonny Bowden, a nutritionist and health author. 'It's very alkalizing for the system,' said the Woodland Hills, Calif. based

91

Bowden, whose books include "Smart Fat" and "The 150 Healthiest Foods on Earth." Having a healthy alkaline balance helps fight germs.'"

Now this confused me. How can lemon – an acidic fruit – alkalinize your system? Body Ecology had exactly what I needed:

"To clear up some of the confusion:

- Acidic and alkaline describe the nature of food *before* it is eaten.

- Acidifying foods and acid-forming foods are the same, making the body more acidic.

- Alkalizing foods and alkaline-forming foods are the same, making the body more alkaline."

I know, now you're wondering what each of these terms mean. So am I...and I thought I knew. I turned to Online Biology Dictionary:

"Acid – a sour-tasting compound that releases hydrogen ions to form a solution with a pH of less than 7, reacts with a base to form a salt, and turns blue litmus red.... An acid solution has a *p*H of less than 7."

I used the same dictionary for the definition of alkaline, which referred me to the definition of alkali.

"Any metallic hydroxide other than ammonia that can join with an acid to form a salt (or with an oil to form soap)."

I didn't find that very helpful so I turned to my old buddy The Merriam-Webster Dictionary:

"a soluble salt obtained from the ashes of plants and consisting largely of potassium or sodium carbonate; *broadly*: a substance (as a hydroxide or carbonate of an alkali metal) having marked basic properties"

Okay, that's a little better, but not much. Let's try this another way. I perused site after site. What I gleaned from these is that lemons are, indeed, acidic before they are eaten, but the body metabolizes them into alkaline. There was plenty of specific science to explain this, but I didn't understand half of it and prefer to keep it simple.

Of course, then I wanted to know why I was even bothering to research this at all. LifeHacks, a new site for me, made it abundantly clear.

1. Gives your immune system a boost.

2. Excellent source of potassium.

3. Aids digestion.

4. Cleanses your system.

5. Freshens your breath.

6. Keeps your skin blemish-free.

7. Helps you lose weight.

8. Reduces inflammation.

9. Gives you an energy boost.

10. Helps to cut out caffeine.

11. Helps fight viral infections.

Now, you do have Chronic Kidney Disease, so be aware that lemons are a high potassium food. Potassium is one of the electrolytes we need to limit. Also, if you are prone to kidney stones, you'll be very interested to know lemons are full of vitamin C, something you may need to avoid.

So far, it sounds like lemon juice in water upon waking is a good thing if you keep the two caveats above in mind but I think I'll just check into this a bit more.

I looked in my first CKD book, *What Is It and How Did I Get It? Early Stage Chronic Kidney Disease*, and discovered this succinct explanation of why you want to keep the potassium levels under guard as a CKD patient:

"Potassium is something you need to limit when you have CKD despite the fact that potassium not only dumps waste from your cells but also helps the kidneys, heart and muscles to function normally. Too much potassium can cause irregular heartbeat and even heart attack. This can be the most immediate danger of not limiting your potassium….

Keep in mind that as you age (you already know I'm in my 60s), your kidneys don't do such a great job of eliminating potassium. So, just by aging, you may have an abundance of potassium. Check your blood tests. 3.5-5 is considered a safe level of potassium. You may have a problem if your blood level of potassium is 5.1-6, and you definitely need to attend to it if it's above 6. Speak to your nephrologist (although he or she will probably bring it up before you do)."

If you're in the normal potassium range on your blood tests as I am, I say go for the lemon juice in water first thing in the morning. Of course, I'm not a doctor and – even if I were – I'm not your doctor, so check with him or her first.

5/23/16 *Apple Cider Vinegar?*

I woke up thinking, 'apple cider vinegar." Granted, that's an odd thought for the first thing in the morning... or is it? Last week, I blogged about the benefits of drinking lemon juice in a glass of water first thing in the morning. Okay, you've read the blog; you know that.

What you may not know is that the blog is posted on a multitude of Facebook chronic illness sites. A reader on one of these sites commented on the blog. I don't remember exactly what she said, but it had something to do with her taking apple cider vinegar every day to help keep her body in alkaline balance.

Ah, now that first thought of the day today is starting to make sense. Monday is blog day for me. It looks like my mind was providing me with a topic for today's blog.

I'll bet the first question you have is why she would want to help keep her body in alkaline balance. Let's do a little back tracking to answer that question. As per last week's blog, Dr. Jonny Bowden, a nutritionist and health author, tells us, "Having a healthy alkaline balance helps fight germs." No contest, I'm sure we all want to do that.

I know, I know, now you'd like to know why alkaline balance – as opposed to acidic body chemistry – does that. I do, too. An article on MedIndia, a respected medical site, explains this:

"A pH of less than 7 is acidic and a pH of more than 7 is alkaline, water being neutral with pH=7. Since one of the most important measurements of health is the pH of the body fluids, it is very important to have an acid-base balance. Any imbalance, especially those leaning towards acidic, could be associated with health disorders including obesity, tiredness, premature aging, heart disease, diabetes and cancer."

Reminder: "The pH of a solution is a measure of the molar concentration of hydrogen ions in the solution and as such is a measure of the acidity or basicity of the solution." Thank you, Hyperphysics for the definition.

Did you catch diabetes in the MedIndia quote? That is the number one cause of Chronic Kidney Disease. This is what I wrote about that in my first CKD book *What Is It and How Did I Get It? Early Stage Chronic Kidney Disease*,

"In fact, the U.S. has the highest rate of CKD with 210 people per million having it, and two thirds of those cases caused by diabetes or HBP."

And that was back in 2011. Two thirds of 210 people per million. .. and we don't know how many of them developed CKD from HBP – or diabetes. Taking no chances, I'll opt for alkaline balance in my body, even though I already have Chronic Kidney Disease.

Next question: how does apple cider vinegar help keep a body in alkaline balance? Let's go back to last week's blog again.

"Body Ecology had exactly what I needed:

'To clear up some of the confusion:

- Acidic and alkaline describe the nature of food *before* it is eaten.

- Acidifying foods and acid-forming foods are the same, making the body more acidic.

- Alkalizing foods and alkaline-forming foods are the same, making the body more alkaline. '"

All right then, we get it that something acidic – like vinegar – could actually be alkaline once it's ingested. And we understand that an alkaline balance can keep us healthier. But we have CKD. Is apple cider vinegar something we can take?

Kidney Hospital China was helpful here, although I am still leery of websites that offer online doctor advice. They maintain that it can lower your blood pressure – a good thing since high blood pressure is not only a cause of CKD, but also can make it worse. They also consider it an anti-inflammatory, although I'm beginning to wonder if all alkaline foods are. Then they mention it helps prevent colds and removes toxins in the blood. Both will help relieve some of the kidney's burden.

This warning was the first I'd seen in all the blogs and natural eating sites I perused for information about today's topic... and it comes from Kidney Hospital China:

"Apple cider vinegar is high in potassium and phosphorus, so kidney disease patients who have high potassium and high phosphorus levels in blood need to avoid the intake of the drinks."

In *The Book of Blogs: Moderate Stage Chronic Kidney Disease, Part 1,* I referred to an article entitled **Vegetarian diet helps kidney disease patients stay healthy** in order to point out why we need to keep our phosphorous levels low:

"Individuals with kidney disease cannot adequately rid the body of phosphorus, which is found in dietary proteins and is a common food additive. Kidney disease patients must limit their phosphorous intake, as high levels of the mineral can lead to heart disease and death."

In *The Book of Blogs: Moderate Stage Chronic Kidney Disease, Part 2,* I succinctly reminded us why we want to watch our potassium intake:

"But isn't potassium good for you? After all, it does help the heart, muscles, and our beloved kidneys function normally as well as dumping wastes from our cells. Here's the kicker, an excess of potassium can cause irregular heartbeat and even heart attack."

All in all, I think this might be a go. Do talk it over with your nephrologist or renal dietician before you start on a regiment of apple cider vinegar. I only research; they've been to medical school. By the way, many of these sites talked about the pleasing taste of this drink. I may have to try it just to see if any drink containing vinegar tastes good.

5/30/16 *Psoriatic Arthritis on Memorial Day*

Today is Memorial Day. I find myself having a hard time saying 'happy' and 'Memorial Day' together. For those of you outside of the U.S., this is a holiday started as Decoration Day by freed slaves after our Civil War to commemorate the lives of those who died earning their freedom. Slowly, individual states made this day for decorating graves a holiday and then it became a national one.

I am married to a veteran. There is nothing happy about this holiday, although there is respect and gratitude... at least in my house.

I have respect and gratitude for our living soldiers, too. That brings us to the subject of today's blog: psoriatic arthritis and Chronic Kidney Disease. A close friend of the family – an Airman – wanted this information for his father. I was happy to oblige him, even more than I usually am to answer readers' questions since he is military and he asked on Memorial Day.

As usual, we need to go back to the basics here. In this case, that means going back to the blog about psoriasis in *The Book of Blogs: Moderate Stage Chronic Kidney Disease, Part 2.* That's where I first wrote the following information about psoriasis:

"...according to Psoriasis.com:

'psoriasis is a chronic (long-lasting) disease of the immune system. While the exact cause of psoriasis is unknown, scientists believe the immune system mistakenly activates a reaction in the skin cells, which speeds up the growth cycle of skin cells.'

There are seven types of psoriasis. The one you are probably familiar with – if you are familiar with any – is plaque psoriasis. WebMD tells us:

"About eight in 10 people with psoriasis have this type. It is also sometimes known as psoriasis vulgaris. Plaque psoriasis causes raised, inflamed, red skin covered by silvery white scales. These may also itch or burn. Plaque psoriasis can appear anywhere on your body…."

Here's the most important information in that particular blog for us as CKD patients:

"…doctors now know they need to screen psoriasis patients for CKD, although it seems to be only those patients with over 3% of their bodies affected by psoriasis who have doubled their risk of CKD. With 60% of the population at risk for CKD, it could be that percentage may change once these routine CKD screenings for psoriasis are in place, especially since psoriasis is also so common among every ethnic group. This, of course, also includes those populations we know are at high risk for CKD."

But my young Airman friend asked about psoriatic arthritis and Chronic Kidney Disease, so we need to take a look at what arthritis is.

According to the U.S. National Library of Medicine:

"Arthritis is a general term for conditions that affect the joints and surrounding tissues. Joints are places in the body where bones come together, such as the knees, wrists, fingers, toes, and hips. The two most common types of arthritis are osteoarthritis and rheumatoid arthritis."

Hmmm, no mention of psoriatic arthritis. That's all right. I'm sure the American College of Rheumatology can help us out here.

"Psoriatic arthritis is a type of inflammation that occurs in about 15 percent of patients who have a skin rash called psoriasis. This particular arthritis can affect any joint in the body, and symptoms vary from person to person. Research has shown that persistent inflammation from psoriatic arthritis can lead to joint damage. Fortunately, available treatments for are effective for most people. Psoriatic arthritis usually appears in people between the ages of 30 to 50, but can begin as early as childhood. Men and women are equally at risk. Children with psoriatic arthritis are also at risk to develop uveitis (inflammation of the middle layer of the eye). Approximately 15 percent of people with psoriasis develop psoriatic arthritis. At times, the arthritis can appear before the skin disorder."

Ah, we know Chronic Kidney Disease is an inflammatory disease. Now we know that arthritis is, too. Being a purist over here, I wanted to check on psoriasis to see if falls into this category, too. Oh my! According to a Position Statement from the American Academy of Dermatologists and AAD Association:

"Psoriasis is a chronic inflammatory, multi-system disease associated with considerable morbidity and co-morbid conditions."

Arthritis is an inflammatory disease; psoriasis is an inflammatory disease; and Chronic Kidney Disease is an inflammatory disease. The common factor here is obvious – inflammatory disease. So what, if anything, can my young Airman friend suggest to his father (other than the most important: See your doctor.)?

Certainly not to take NSAIDS. I defined – and cautioned against – NSAIDS in the glossary of *What Is It and How Did I Get It? Early Stage Chronic Kidney Disase*. There's been no new research to debunk this warning since then.

"**NSAID:** Non-steroidal anti-inflammatory drugs such as ibuprofen, aspirin, Aleve or naproxen usually used for arthritis or pain management, can worsen kidney disease, sometimes irreversibly."

Well, what can the man do for these three inflammatory diseases? Let's take a look at Dr. Rich Snyder's guest blog in *The Book of Blogs: Moderate Stage Chronic Kidney Disease, Part 1.* In discussing probiotics and alkaline water, he threw in this little gem.

"Alkaline/anti-inflammatory based diet: Some say, "Eat for your blood type." But, what is the DASH diet for hypertension? It is not just a low salt. It is also full of antioxidants and anti-inflammatory."

Food as medicine for an inflammatory body condition? DASH diet? What is the DASH diet? "DASH stands for Dietary Approaches to Stop Hypertension...."

Take a look at the Mayo Clinic's information about this. There's far too much to explore here, but I do urge you to remember you have CKD, so although it is an inflammatory disease, you need to be mindful of your renal diet should you decide to adopt the DASH diet.

6/6/16 *Two Levels?*

I am now the very satisfied user of a Bi-level Positive Airway Pressure Machine (BiPAP). I fought against this for years, preferring to use a Mandibular Advancement Device (MAD) instead so I wouldn't be 'tethered' to a machine. After only two nights of sleeping with the Bi-PAP, I have more energy and less brain fog. Heck, that happened after only one night. I wonder just how much of the low energy and high brain fog that I was attributing to Chronic Kidney Disease was really from not enough oxygen and too much CO2 in my lungs.

Whoops, here I am jumping in at the end again. Maybe a reminder of what a MAD is would be the logical place to start. This is what I wrote in *The Book of Blogs: Moderate Stage Chronic Kidney Disease, Part 2*, "...the MAD forces your airway open by advancing your lower jaw or mandibular."

If your air passages are restricted, you're simply not getting enough air into the lungs.

After well over two years, my sleep apnea started becoming worse instead of better, even when the MAD had been extended as far as it could go to keep that airway open. (Laughing over here; it sounds like an instrument of torture. It isn't.)

You're probably wondering what this has to do with CKD. I used my baby, *What Is It and How Did I Get it? Early Stage Chronic Kidney Disease* to find out.

"The first mention of the lungs was in an explanation of your nephrologist's ROS. 'Then came the Review of Systems [ROS]. …, the lungs were referred to with questions about coughs, shortness of breath and dyspnea.'"

That does still leave us with the question of why the lungs were covered at all in this examination for CKD. According one of the National Institutes of Health's sites, sleep apnea can raise blood pressure, which in itself is one of the problems of CKD. It can also result in glomerular hyperfiltration. The chart below is from their site. Notice 'eGFR declines' is one of the results. These three areas are the most important to us as CKD patients, which doesn't mean the other effects should be ignored.

What was missing for me was why it was so important to get as much air into the lungs as possible. Livescience's site was able to help me out here.

"….The lungs are responsible for removing oxygen from the air we breathe and transferring it to our blood where it can be sent to our cells. The lungs also remove carbon dioxide, which we exhale."

Why not a Continuous Positive Airway Pressure (CPAP) machine then, you ask? WebMD explains:

"A CPAP machine increases air pressure in your throat so that your airway doesn't collapse when you breathe in."

Got it... and necessary when you have sleep apnea. So the next logical question is why was I prescribed a BiPAP instead. Notice in the explanation from Livescience above that the lungs also remove carbon dioxide. Yep, not enough was being removed as I slept.

I liked this explanation of the difference between the CPAP and the BiPAP from verywell :

"The key distinguishing feature of BiPAP is that the pressurized air is delivered at two alternating levels. The inspiratory positive airway pressure (IPAP) is higher and supports a breath as it is taken in. Conversely, the ex-piratory positive airway pressure (EPAP) is a lower pres-sure that allows you to breathe out. These pressures are preset based on a prescription provided by your sleep doctor and alternate just like your breathing pattern."

It's when you breathe out that you rid yourself of car-bon dioxide. But I wanted to know why too much of that in your system is not a good thing. I was delighted to find this scientific, yet understandable, (albeit older) posting by then Ph.D. candidate Shannon DeVaney on MadSci, which is a service provided by Washington University in St. Louis.

"...much of the body's excess carbon dioxide ends up in the blood.... The net effect of increased carbon dioxide in the blood is lowered blood pH (that is, the blood be-comes more acidic). The ability of hemoglobin to bind with oxygen decreases with decreasing pH in a phenomenon called the Bohr effect (sic). Because of the Bohr effect, increasing CO_2 concentrations indirectly reduce the oxygen carrying capacity of the blood.

Carbon dioxide can also react with parts of the hemoglobin molecule to form carbamino compounds. The formation of these compounds directly reduces the ability of hemoglobin to bind with oxygen and therefore also reduces the oxygen carrying capacity of the blood.

So, in these two ways (indirectly by reducing blood pH and directly by reacting with hemoglobin) carbon dioxide can reduce the ability of our blood to carry oxygen to tissues throughout the body where it is needed. It's a good thing, then, that the excess carbon dioxide in our blood diffuses into our lungs, where it leaves the body when we exhale."

Except in my case, it wasn't. Hence the BiPAP to help me out. If the results of the last two nights continue, it seems I needed an awful lot of helping out... and I didn't know it. So far today, I have booked a combined 70th birthday cruise to Cuba for Bear and me, conferred many times by phone and text with my wonderful sister-in-law – Judy Peck (mentioned several times in *SlowItDownCKD 2015*) – about cabins, insurance, land excursions, packages, etc., then gotten back to our travel agent with our decisions, spoken with three different doctors and two labs, communicated with three of my daughters, contacted our donation center for pick up, and scheduled several maintenance jobs for my house – and I'm not tired. I haven't yawned once. I could learn to like living like this.

By the way, between Medicare and my secondary in-surance, this is not costing me a thing. Oh goody, more money for our birthday present to ourselves.

6/13/16 *Connected*

Full Definition of connected from the Merriam-Webster Dictionary

1: joined or linked together

2: having the parts or elements logically linked togeth-er *<presented a thoroughly connected view of the prob-lem>*

3: related by blood or marriage

4: having social, professional, or commercial relation-ships *<a well-connected lawyer>*

5: of a set: having the property that any two of its points can be joined by a line completely contained in the set; also: incapable of being separated into two or more closed disjoint subsets

Growing up in New York, I often heard the word used to suggest someone was associated with the Mafia. You know, like you see in gangster movies. But, that's not what today's blog is about. It's about the connec-tion among all the chronic ailments you have. That would be the second definition.

Before we start, I need to remind you that I'm not a doctor and have never claimed to be one. This is my thinking from my research. This blog was sparked by a conversation on the Facebook page
Stage 3 'n 4 CKD Kidneybeaners Gathering Place in

which Robin Rose got me to thinking about the connection between CKD and inflammation. Maybe it will give you something to think about, too.

PubMed, part of the U.S. National Library of Medicine, tells us:

"Inflammation is the response of the vasculature or tissues to various stimuli. An acute and chronic pro-inflammatory state exists in patients with chronic kidney disease (CKD), contributing substantially to morbidity and mortality. ... Inflammation contributes to the progression of CKD by inducing the release of cytokines and the increased production and activity of adhesion molecules, which together contribute to T cell adhesion and migration into the interstitium, subsequently attracting pro-fibrotic factors. Inflammation in CKD also causes mortality from cardiovascular disease by contributing to the development of vascular calcifications and endothelial dysfunction. ... "

In that one quotation, you have the definition of inflammation and its causes. I thought I'd try easing into this difficult explanation.

In *The Book of Blogs: Moderate Stage Chronic Kidney Disease, Part 1*, I accepted the connection, but without thought:

"And to answer your question about what colon cancer has to do with Chronic Kidney Disease, you have to remember you are medically compromised already. Cancer is a disease caused by inflammation, just as Chronic Kidney Disease is."

That's two chronic diseases caused by inflammation: CKD and colon cancer. There are more, many more.

By the time I wrote *The Book of Blogs: Moderate Stage Chronic Kidney Disease, Part 2*, I was aware that sinusitis is another inflammatory disease.

"According to Canada.com:

'The narrowed nasal passageway caused by a deviated septum can cause mucus to become blocked by preventing the drainage of mucus from a sinus into the nasal cavity. Excess mucus inside the sinuses presents an attractive environment for bacteria, leading to a sinus infection. This in turn causes inflammation of the sinuses (sinusitis), and because it can happen regularly, chronic sinusitis can occur.'"

That's three chronic diseases caused by inflammation: CKD, colon cancer, and sinusitis. But there are more, many more.

Last year, I wrote *SlowItDownCKD 2015* and included this information:

"Another standby, WebMD, explains:

'Bladder infections are known as cystitis or inflammation of the bladder. They are common in women, but very rare in men. More than half of all women get at least one bladder infection at some time in their lives. However, a man's chance of getting cystitis increases as he ages, due to in part to an increase in prostate size....

Bladder infections are not serious if treated right away. But they tend to come back in some people. Rarely, this can lead to kidney infections, which are more serious and may result in permanent kidney damage. So it's very important to treat the underlying causes of a bladder infection and to take preventive steps to keep them from coming back."

Oh, so repeated bladder infections can lead to kidney infections, although rarely.'"

That's four diseases caused by inflammation: CKD, colon cancer, sinusitis, and cystitis. But there are more, many more.

According to MedicineNet at:

"Psoriasis is a noncontagious skin condition that produces plaques of thickened, scaling skin. The dry flakes of skin scales are thought to result from the excessively rapid proliferation of skin cells triggered by inflammatory chemicals produced by specialized white blood cells called lymphocytes. Psoriasis commonly affects the skin of the elbows, knees, and scalp."

That's five diseases caused by inflammation: CKD, colon cancer, sinusitis, cystitis, and psoriasis. But there are more, many more.

Let's not forget arthritis.

According to last year's article in *Blood Purification Journal,*

"Chronic inflammation should be regarded as a common comorbid condition in CKD and especially in dialysis patients. A number of interventions have been proven to be safe and effective in well-designed clinical studies. This includes such inexpensive approaches as modification of physical activity and dietary supplementation. "

6/20/16 *A Cautionary Tale*

Last week, I found myself crushed for time: a friend was coming to visit from Florida, we had a Father's Day brunch at our house, there were theater tickets, one of the kids needed immediate aid since she was in her own time crunch, the list goes on and on. Taking that into account and not wanting to add that old demon 'stress' to the list, I thought I'd do a quick, easy blog about acupuncture/acupressure and Chronic Kidney Disease.

But while researching I discovered a number of sites with online doctors and changed my topic immediately. The ones I clicked on were:

- Health Tap Inc. [US]

- Kidneyfailureweb.com

- Kidney-treatment.org

- CKDstage.com

- KidneyABC.com

- KidneyServiceChina.org

- Kidney-support.org.

I'm sure there are more, but rather than be an alarmist, I want to be an explainer.

Explainer of what you ask. Not acupuncture or acupressure. There's a discussion of how acupressure works in the May 4th blog in *SlowItDownCKD 2015*. Acupuncture works on the same principle, but using very fine needles rather than pressure. I happily and confidently made use of both before my CKD diagnose and only ceased my treatments when the senior acupuncturist working on me told me these treatments would not help with the CKD. That was over nine years ago. He may have changed his opinion since then.

I want to explain why online doctors are not such a great idea. I can practically see some of you rolling your eyes at me while others are thinking, "Why not?" Okay, maybe they're legal, but are they ethical? I found a fairly straight forward abstract on ResearchGate which states:

"...online medical consultations pose greater dangers to patients compared to traditional off-line consultations.... while new technologies may aid doctors in making better diagnoses at a distance, they often bring new concerns."

I find myself struggling here. I am all in favor of online doctor summaries by your doctors, test reports from your labs, and general medication explanations from the internet. However, I simply cannot understand how someone who has never met you, someone who has not examined your body, someone who has never spoken with you can advise you on your health.

I've mentioned before that I have psoriasis, arthritis, neuropathy, sleep apnea, and probably a host of other as-yet-undiagnosed-inflammatory based diseases (This might be a good time to reread last week's blog about inflammation caused disease: *Connected.*) How can someone who's never met me take all of this into account when dealing with my health?

A perfect example of what I'm talking about is from the IMPRESSIONS section of my rheumatologist's recent report,

"This is a very complex patient that presents today with generalized myalgias and arthralgia....Her health history is complicated by carpal tunnel syndrome, neuropathy and chronic kidney disease, stage 3."

She has not missed a trick. Myalgia, according to the Medical Dictionary is muscular pain. The Mayo Clinic tells us arthralgia is joint pain. So my muscles and joints hurt. Without seeing me, without testing my joints and muscles, without seeing if the joints are disfigured or the muscles flaccid (for example) how could she help me?

I'm not one to take pain killers, especially NSAIDS which are defined in the glossary of *What Is It and How Did I Get It? Early Stage Chronic Kidney Disease.*

"NSAID: Non-steroidal anti-inflammatory drugs such as ibuprofen, aspirin, Aleve or naproxen usually used for arthritis or pain management, can worsen kidney disease, sometimes irreversibly."

So I have pain and I can tolerate it. I can't help but wonder what an online doctor would diagnose. I decided to become a test case. I contacted an online doctor from one of the sites listed above. This is the transcript of that online chat, errors and all.

"Welcome! This is a real online-doctor, not a robort. If you have any questions on kidney disease, feel free to type your questions, you will surely get reply. No consultation fee.

If the online doctors are all busy and you can't get response for a long time, you can contact us by phone or email. (Contact information followed.)

renal-onlinedoctor: Hello, I am renal-onlinedoctor, I am very glad to talk with you!

You: I have pain. What do I do about it?

renal-onlinedoctor: hello, your age and gender?

You: 69 female

renal-onlinedoctor: ok, what is the current kidney function or creatinine level? do you know

You: 50%

renal-onlinedoctor: ok, Any symptoms? foamy urine, swelling, fatigue, back pain, anemia, itching, etc

You: Just joint and muscle pain.

renal-onlinedoctor: i see. Do you have Diabetes, high blood pressure, or other problem?

You: HBP, neuropathy, arthritis, psoriasis

renal-onlinedoctor: ok, What are the current medicines or treatment?

You: Only hbp meds and arthritis meds.

renal-onlinedoctor: okay i see. I'd like to send you re-lated info and advice. What is your Email address?

At this point, I ended the chat since I thought I might be deluged with emails if I responded. Have I proven any-thing? Only that the online portion of dealing with an online doctor is extremely general.

Where are the questions about my weight? As I wrote in *The Book of Blogs: Moderate Stage Chronic Kidney Disease, Part 2:*

"Keeping your weight down is one of the ways to help retard the progression of the disease. How? By not al-lowing yourself to become obese. Obviously, if you keep gaining weight, you can become obese. Obesity is one of the contributing factors for developing diabetes. Diabetes may lead to, and complicates, the treatment of, CKD."

And what about exercise? In *The Book of Blogs: Moderate Stage Chronic Kidney Disease, Part 1,* I included the following from the American Kidney Fund:

"Exercise can help you stay healthy. To get the most benefit, exercise for at least 30 minutes, 5 days of the week."

Yes, it is possible the online doctor may have included such information in the emails (s)he wanted to send me, but how specific to my unique, complex medical situation would they have been... or how specific to yours?

6/27/16 *Bridging the Gap...*

Which gap? The anion. What's that, you say.

"The anion gap deals with the body's acidity. A high reading for the anion gap could indicate renal failure."

That's what I wrote in *What Is It and How Did I Get It? Early Stage Chronic Kidney Disease.* But you know what? It's just not enough information any more. Why? I'm glad you asked. Oh, by the way, if you want to check your own reading look in the Comprehensive Metabolic Panel part of your blood tests, but only if your doctor requested it be tested.

I mentioned a few blogs back that I returned to a rheu-matologist I hadn't seen in years and she chose to treat me as a new patient. Considering how much had hap-pened medically since I'd last seen her, that made sense to me and I agreed to blood tests, an MRI, and a bone density test.

The only reading that surprised me was an abnormally high one for anion gap. The acceptable range is 4 – 18. My reading was 19. While I have Chronic Kidney Dis-ease, my kidneys have not failed (Thank goodness and my hard work.) In addition, I've become quite aware of just how important acidity and alkaline states are and have been dealing with this, although apparently not effectively.

MedFriendly – a new site for me written by Dr. Dominic Carone for the express purpose of simplifying complex medical terms for the lay person – explains it this way:

"…. Too high of an anion gap level can mean that there is acidosis (too much acid in the blood) due to diabetes mellitus. The high anion gap level can also be due to lactic acidosis, in which the high level of acid is due a buildup of a substance called lactic acid. … A high anion gap can also be due to drug poisoning or kidney failure. …When the anion gap is high, further tests are usually needed to diagnose the cause of the problem."

Ah, I remember writing a bit about acidosis in *The Book of Blogs: Moderate Stage Chronic Kidney Disease, Part 1.* It had to do with fruits and vegetables.

"'After three years, consuming fruits and vegetables or taking the oral medication reduced a marker of metabolic acidosis and preserved kidney function to similar extents. Our findings suggest that an apple a day keeps the nephrologist away,' study author Dr. Nimrit Goraya, of Texas A&M College of Medicine, said in a university news release."

Apparently, some CKD suffers have metabolic systems that are severely acidic. Fruits and vegetables are highly alkaline. This may counteract the acidity in the patients mentioned above AND those that have less metabolic acidosis (acid in the body).

Okay, I like fruit and I like vegetables. Ummm, will my limitation of three servings of each within the kidney friendly fruit and vegetable lists do the trick, I wonder. Looks like I'll be questioning both the rheumatologist and the renal dietician about that.

Recently I've written about alkaline being the preferred state of a CKD patient's body. That is the antithesis of an acid body state. Years ago, Dr. Richard Synder was a guest blogger here and also interviewed me on his radio show. He is the author of **What You Must Know about Kidney Disease** and a huge proponent of alkaline water. Here's what he had to say about that (also from *Part 1*):

"I have taken alkaline water myself and I notice a difference in how I feel. Our bodies are sixty percent water. Why would I not want to put the best type of water into it? Mineralized water helps with bone health. In alkalinized water, the hydroxyl ions produced from the reaction of the bicarbonate and the gastric acid with a low pH produce more hydroxyl ions which help buffer the acidity we produce on a daily basis. (Me interrupting here: During our visit last Monday, I noticed that my extremely health conscious, non-CKD, Florida friend drinks this.)

Where are these buffers? In the bones and in the cells, as well as some extracellular buffers. You are helping lower the total body acidity and decreasing the inflammation brought on by it. You do this early on so that you don't have a problem with advanced acidosis later. Why wait until you are acidotic before doing something?"

Notice his comment about lowering body acidity and decreasing inflammation. We already know CKD is an inflammatory disease. There was something to this. I went back to *The Book of Blogs: Moderate Stage Chronic Kidney Disease, Part 2* to tease it out.

"'Belly fat is also much more inflammatory than fat located elsewhere in the body and can create its own inflammatory chemicals (as a tumor would).

Inflammatory? Isn't CKD an inflammatory disease? I went to The National Center for Biotechnology Information, which took me to the National Library of Medicine and finally to a National Institute of Health study for the answer.

'The persistent inflammatory state is common in diabetes and Chronic Kidney Disease (CKD).

This is a lot to take in at once. What it amounts to is that another way to possibility prevent the onset of CKD is to lower your phosphorous intake so that you don't accumulate belly fat.'"

Phosphorous? Once we have CKD, we do have phosphorous restrictions. But I have never had high phosphorous readings. Maybe I should be exploring an abundance of lactic acid as a cause of the high anion gap reading instead.

According to Heathline.com,

"Lactic acidosis occurs when there's too much lactic acid in your body. Many things can cause a buildup of lactic acid. These include chronic alcohol use, heart failure, cancer, seizures, liver failure, prolonged lack of oxygen, and low blood sugar. Even prolonged exercise can lead to lactic acid buildup."

I'm definitely barking up the wrong tree here.

Wait a minute. I recently started using a BiPAP since I have sleep apnea and wasn't exhaling enough CO2. That could cause acidosis, but it would be respiratory acidosis. Say, a basic metabolic panel would expose that. Nope, that's not it either since my CO2 levels were normal.

It looks like this is going to be one of those blogs that asks more questions than it answers. I do have an appointment with the rheumatologist on the 20[th]and will ask for answers then.

7/4/16 *We, the People Who Have CKD...*

Happy Independence Day! Here in the United States, we usually celebrate with fireworks and bar-b-ques that may include renal friendly foods, at least at my house. We take our pets inside and try to shield them from the sounds of the fireworks that make them so uncomfortable and then we try to enjoy the heat, the sun, and the parades.

I'm all for Independence Day celebrations, but shy away from them myself. I'm like our pets; I can do without the noise. Since getting older (or medically 'elderly,' which always gives me a giggle), I can also do without the heat and the crowds. We used to have renal friendly bar-b-ques at our house, but now our kids are older and visit fiancés, go to bachelorette weekend celebrations, or go camping in other states during this long holiday weekend.

And I realize I do not want to be that far from what is euphemistically called a 'restroom' here in Arizona for all that long. There could be many reasons for that, my elderly state (Humph!); a urinary tract infection (UTI); a weak bladder; or interstitial cystitis.

A reader and good online friend – another Texas connection, by the way – asked me to write about interstitial cystitis today. There seems to be some confusion among us – meaning Chronic Kidney Disease patients – between chronic UTIs and interstitial cystitis.

UTI is a descriptive term we probably all know since we have CKD and have to be aware of them. We have to be careful they don't spread to the bladder and, eventually (but rarely), to the kidneys. That can cause even more kidney damage. I explained a bit more in *The Book of Blogs: Moderate Stage Chronic Kidney Disease, Part 2*:

"The second nephrologist to treat me referred me to an urologist when he realized I was on my fifth UTI in the same summer and he suspected this one had spread to my bladder. The urologist actually had me look through the cystoscope (I'm adding this today: a sort of long, narrow tube inserted to view both the urethra and bladder) myself to reassure me that the lower urinary tract infection had not spread to the upper urinary tract where the bladder is located."

We know we have to be vigilant. That's where interstitial cystitis comes in. Let's take a look at *SlowItDownCKD 2015* for more information about cystitis:

"Another standby, WebMD, explains:

'Bladder infections are known as cystitis or inflammation of the bladder. They are common in women, but very rare in men. More than half of all women get at least one bladder infection at some time in their lives. However, a man's chance of getting cystitis increases as he ages, due to in part to an increase in prostate size....

Bladder infections are not serious if treated right away. But they tend to come back in some people. Rarely, this can lead to kidney infections, which are more serious and may result in permanent kidney damage. So it's very important to treat the underlying causes of a bladder infection and to take preventive steps to keep them from coming back.'"

Okay so we get the cystitis part of the condition, but what does interstitial mean? MedicineNet defines it this way:

"Pertaining to being between things, especially between things that are normally closely spaced. The word interstitial is much used in medicine and has specific meaning, depending on the context. For instance, interstitial cystitis is a specific type of inflammation of the bladder wall."

Hang on, just one more definition. This one is from the Mayo Clinic.

"Interstitial cystitis (in-tur-STISH-ul sis-TIE-tis) — also called painful bladder syndrome — is a chronic condition in which you experience bladder pressure, bladder pain and sometimes pelvic pain, ranging from mild discomfort to severe pain. Your bladder is a hollow, muscular organ that stores urine. The bladder expands until it's full and then signals your brain that it's time to urinate, communicating through the pelvic nerves. This creates the urge to urinate for most people. With interstitial cystitis, these signals get mixed up — you feel the need to urinate more often and with smaller volumes of urine than most people...."

Hmmm, then this is clearly not a UTI. So why do we have to be careful about it? Time to look at the causes – or not. According to the National Institute of Diabetes, Digestive, and Kidney Diseases,

"Researchers are working to understand the causes of IC/PBS and to find effective treatments.

...Scientists believe IC/PBS may be a bladder manifestation of a more general condition that causes inflammation in various organs and parts of the body."

* IC means interstitial cystitis; PBS is painful bladder syndrome

Maybe we should be looking at the cure instead – or not. "At this time there is no cure for interstitial cystitis (IC)." But ichelp.org does mention a number of possible treatments, some of which we cannot use as CKD patients since they may harm the kidneys.

Whoa! No definitive cause, no cure, and treatments which may harm our kidneys. Where's the good news in this? Take another look at the information from The National Institute of Diabetes, Digestive, and Kidney Diseases again. Notice the word 'inflammation'?

Bingo. CKD is also an inflammatory disease and may be that "more general condition that causes inflammation in various organs and parts of the body." Wait, I just remembered this from *The Book of Blogs: Moderate Stage Chronic Kidney Disease, Part 1:*

"Cancer is a disease caused by inflammation, just as Chronic Kidney Disease is. By the way, it's said that al-kaline foods are a better way of eating should cancer rear its ugly head in your life."

So it all comes back to inflammation. Say, didn't I re-cently write a blog about acidity vs. alkaline and in-flammation? Now there's a good way to avoid the heat, the sun, and the parades of Independence Day. Stay inside (maybe while someone is bar-b-quing renal friendly food outside) and peruse old blog posts.

7/11/16 *What's Your Type?*

Every Sunday night, I take a blues dance lesson taught by my daughter, Abby Wegerski, as Sustainable Blues, Phoenix and stay to dance to the music of the live band – for a while. Last week, my good buddy, Karla Lodge, organized a fund raiser. I like to support Karla in whatever she does, so I decided to push myself and go to the fundraiser (a half hour drive each way) after dancing.

To make it even more fun, Bill Weber, the creator of Avery's World, was in from Los Angeles visiting a relative in Tucson. They drove up to Scottsdale to join us at the fundraiser. Now that you've been introduced to some of the people and events in my life, forget them. Here's the important part: as we were having dinner, my Chronic Kidney Disease Awareness Advocacy came up. Bill's relative lit up. It turns out someone very close to her is a transplantee. Her first question to me: What's your blood type?

I explained I was in the moderate stages of CKD and not anywhere near transplant, but she insisted it was very important to know your blood type when you have CKD. She didn't know why. I didn't know why...so that's the subject of today's blog.

Here I am starting in the middle again. We all have a blood type. That's fairly common knowledge, but what exactly are blood types? We'll go about this a bit differently by defining blood group, which is a synonym for blood type. To paraphrase a song we used to sing during the two times I went to a two week stint at summer camp on a farm, "I know because the dictionary tells me so." In this case it's the Merriam-Webster Dictionary:

"one of the classes (as those designated A, B, AB, or O) into which individuals or their blood can be separated on the basis of the presence or absence of specific antigens in the blood —called also *blood type*"

For those of you who are wondering, an antigen is something that's introduced to the body and causes the body to produce antibodies (Think germs). As an undergraduate in good old Hunter College of The City University of New York I learned that 'anti' is a prefix meaning against. 'Gen' is a root which means causing something to happen. Got it. An antigen causes something to happen against something else. In this case, your red blood cells.

I see a hand raised in the back of the room. (This does remind me of when I was teaching college out here in Arizona.) Why are there four types you ask? Good question. Anyone have the answer? I don't either, so let's look it up together. Look! The Smithsonian Institute sums it up in one sentence: "But why humans and apes have these blood types is still a scientific mystery." Now I don't feel so uninformed that I couldn't answer the question. Where, oh where, is Bones when you need her?

Did you know there are numerous other blood groups, too? Usually people don't – unless they happen to be a member of one of them. You should know that your blood type is inherited.

Again, why is it important to know your blood group? Thank you to Disabled World for the following chart, which demonstrates the answer.

They also offer a simple explanation of why blood groups are so important:

"Blood types are very important when a blood transfusion is necessary. In a blood transfusion, a patient must receive a blood type compatible with his or her own blood type. If the blood types are not compatible, red blood cells will clump together, making clots that can block blood vessels and cause death.

If two different blood types are mixed together, the blood cells may begin to clump together in the blood vessels, causing a potentially fatal situation. Therefore, it is important that blood types be matched before blood transfusions take place. In an emergency, type O blood can be given because it is most likely to be accepted by all blood types. However, there is still a risk involved."

As a CKD patient for the last nine years, I have never needed a blood transfusion. Come to think of it, I've never needed one in my almost 70 years on this planet. But that's not to say I may not need one sometime in the future... or that you might not need one. But I'm interested in why it's especially important to know your blood type as a moderate stage CKD patient.

I scoured *What Is It and How Did I Get It? Early Stage Chronic Kidney Disease*, *The Book of Blogs: Moderate Stage Chronic Kidney Disease – Part 1*, *The Book of Blogs: Moderate Stage Chronic Kidney Disease – Part 2*, and *SlowItDownCKD 2015*. Although there is abundant discussion of how the kidneys filter the blood, why their effectiveness in this filtering diminishes in CKD and the production of red blood cells, there is no mention of blood type in any of the books.

I'm beginning to wonder if Bill's relative meant that knowing your blood type is important in general, not especially if you have CKD. Karla, a Physician's Assistant, was strangely quiet during this part of the discussion. I attributed that to her being pre-occupied with the fundraiser she was running... maybe that wasn't the reason.

Although I didn't find the answer to my question, I did run across some intriguing theories during my research. I'm not endorsing them since I know so little about them, simply offering you the information.

The Blood Type Diet (I do remember a colleague being interested in this one about a decade ago.)

Blood Type and Your Personality

7/18/16 *The American Kidney Fund Blog*

I was honored that The American Kidney Fund asked me to write a blog for them. This is that blog. Once it was published last Thursday, I started thinking. If you share the blog and ask those you shared with to share it, too, and they asked their friends to share it, too... imagine how many people would become aware of Chronic Kidney Disease. Will you do that?

Slowing Down CKD—It Can Be Done

When a new family doctor told me nine years ago that I had a problem with my kidneys—maybe chronic kidney disease (CKD)–my first reaction was to demand, "What is it and how did I get it?"

No doctor had ever mentioned CKD before.

I was diagnosed at stage 3; there are only 5 stages. I had to start working to slow it down immediately. I wanted to know how medication, diet, exercise and other lifestyle changes could help. I didn't want to be told what to do without an explanation as to why... and when I couldn't get an explanation that was acceptable to me, I started researching.

I read just about every book I could find concerning this problem. Surprisingly, very few books dealt with the early or moderate stages of the disease. Yet these are the stages when we are most shocked, confused, and maybe even depressed—and the stages at which we have a workable chance of doing something to slow down the progression in the decline of our kidney function.

I've learned that 31 million people—14 percent of the population—have CKD, but most don't know they have it. Many, like me, never experienced any noticeable symptoms. Many, like me, may have had high blood pressure (hypertension) for years before it was diagnosed. Yet, high blood pressure and diabetes are the two leading causes of CKD.

I saw a renal dietician who explained to me how hard protein is on the kidneys... as is phosphorous... and potassium... and, of course, sodium. Out went my daily banana—too high in potassium. Out went restaurant burgers—larger than my daily allowance of protein. Chinese food? Pizza? Too high in sodium. I embraced an entirely new way of eating because it was one of the keys to keeping my kidneys functioning in stage 3.

Another critical piece of slowing down CKD is medication. I was already taking meds to lower my blood pressure when I was first diagnosed with CKD. Two more prescriptions have been added to this in the last nine years: a diuretic that lowers my body's absorption of salt to help prevent fluid from building up in my body (edema), and a drug that widens the blood vessels by relaxing them.

For a very short time, I was also taking a drug to control my pre-diabetes, but my doctor and I achieved the same effects by changing my diet even more. (Bye-bye, sugars and most carbs.) The funny thing is now my favorite food is salad with extra virgin olive oil and balsamic vinegar. I never thought that would happen: I was a chocoholic!

Exercise, something I loved until my arthritis got in the way, was also important. I used to dance vigorously several nights a week; now it's once a week with weights, walking, and a stationary bike on the other days. I think I took sleep for granted before CKD, too, and I now make it a point to get a good night's sleep each day. A sleep apnea device improved my sleep—and my kidney function rose another two points.

I realized I needed to rest, too. Instead of giving a lecture, running to an audition, and coming home to meet a deadline, I slowly started easing off until I didn't feel like I was running on empty all the time. I ended up happily retiring from both acting and teaching at a local college, giving me more time to work on my CKD awareness advocacy.

I was sure others could benefit from all the research I had done and all I had learned, so I wrote my first book, *What Is It and How Did I Get It? Early Stage Chronic Kidney Disease*, in 2011. I began a blog after a nephrologist in India told me he wanted his newly diagnosed patients to read my book, but most of them couldn't afford the bus fare to the clinic, much less a book. I published each chapter as a blog post. The nephrologist translated my posts, printed them and distributed them to his patients—who took the printed copies back to their villages. I now have readers in 106 different countries who ask me questions I hadn't even thought of. I research for them and respond with a blog post, reminding them to speak with their nephrologists and/or renal nutritionists before taking any action... and that I'm not a doctor.

Each time I research, I'm newly amazed at how much there is to learn about CKD...and how many tools can help slow it down. Diet is the obvious one. But if you smoke or drink, stop, or at least cut down. If you don't exercise, start. Adequate, good quality sleep is another tool. Don't underestimate rest either; you're not being lazy when you rest, you're preserving whatever kidney function you have left. I am not particularly a pill person, but if there's a medication prescribed that will slow down the gradual decline of my kidney function, I'm all for it.

My experience proves that you can slow down CKD. I was diagnosed at stage 3 and I am still there, nine years later. It takes knowledge, commitment, and discipline—but it can be done, and it's worth the effort. I'm sneaking up on 70 now and know this is where I want to spend my energy for the rest of my life: chronic kidney disease awareness advocacy. I think it's just that important.

SlowItDownCKD is the umbrella under which Gail Rae-Garwood writes her CKD books and blog, offers talks, participates in book signings, is interviewed on podcasts and radio shows, and writes guest blogs. Her website is *www.gail-raegarwood.com.*

7/24/16 *Hair Today, Gone Tomorrow (Heaven Forbid)*

I have noticed my hair coming out in alarming amounts when I wash it in the shower. At first, I thought, "I don't brush it so this must be the way I shed dead hairs." Sure, Gail, keep telling yourself that. I have always had a glorious mane. No more. You can see more and more of my scalp with each shower. OMG!

I've read pleas for help from Chronic Kidney Disease patients about just this issue...but they were dialysis patients. I'm Stage 3, more often with a GFR in the low 50s rather than the low 30s. Could it be my Chronic Kidney Disease causing the hair loss – I'll feel better if we called it 'hair thinning' – or simply my almost seventy decades on Earth?

I can appreciate those of you asking, "Her what is in the low 50s?" Let's take a peek at *What Is It and How Did I Get It? Early Stage Chronic Kidney Disease* for a definition of GFR.

"**GFR:** Glomerular filtration rate [if there is a lower case "e" before the term, it means estimated glomerular filtration rate] which determines both the stage of kidney disease and how well the kidneys are functioning."

Of course, now you want to know, and rightfully so, what those numbers mean. In *The Book of Blogs: Moderate Stage Chronic Kidney Disease, Part 2*, I included a helpful chart from DaVita along with some of my own comments which explains.

"Think of the stages as a test with 100 being the highest score. These are the stages and their treatments:

STAGE 1: (normal or high) – above 90 – usually requires watching, not treatment, although many people decide to make life style changes now: following a renal diet, exercising, lowering blood pressure, ceasing to smoke, etc.

 STAGE 2: (mild) – 60-89 – Same as for stage one

STAGE 3A: (moderate) – 45-59 – This is when you are usually referred to a nephrologist (kidney specialist). You'll need a renal (kidney) dietitian, too, since you need to be rigorous in avoiding more than certain amounts of protein, potassium, phosphorous, and sodium in your diet to slow down the deterioration of your kidneys. Each patient has different needs so there is no one diet. The diet is based on your lab results. Medications such as those for high blood pressure may be prescribed to help preserve your kidney function.

STAGE 3B: (moderate) – 30-44 – same as above, except the patient may experience symptoms.

STAGE 4: (severe 15-29) – Here's when dialysis may start. A kidney transplant may be necessary instead of dialysis (artificial cleansing of your blood). Your nephrologist will probably want to see you every three months and request labs before each visit.

STAGE 5: (End stage) – below 15 – Dialysis or transplant is necessary to continue living."

As for the hair itself, I wondered what it's made of so I started googling and came up with Hilda Sustaita, Department Chair of Cosmetology at Houston Community College – Northwest's, definition.

"Hair is made of protein which originates in the hair follicle. As the cells mature, they fill up with a fibrous protein called keratin. These cells lose their nucleus and die as they travel up the hair follicle. Approximately 91 percent of the hair is protein made up of long chains of amino acids."

Uh-oh, Chronic Kidney Disease patients need to lower their protein intake. I'm constantly talking about my five ounce daily limitation. I remembered quoting something about protein limitation in *The Book of Blogs: Moderate Stage Chronic Kidney Disease, Part 1* and so looked for that quote. This is what I found.

"This is part of an article from one of DaVita's sites.

… Depending on what stage of Chronic Kidney Disease you're in, your renal dietitian will adjust the amounts of protein, sodium, phosphorus and potassium in your diet. … The CKD non-dialysis diet includes calculated amounts of high quality protein. Damaged kidneys have a difficult time getting rid of protein waste products, so cutting back on non-essential protein will put less stress on your kidneys."

But I have friends near my age without CKD whose hair is thinning, too. They're not on protein restricted diets, so what's causing their hair thinning?

According to WebMD,

"'The diameter of the hair shaft diminishes as we get older,' explains Zoe Draelos, M.D., clinical associate professor of dermatology at Wake Forest University School of Medicine. That means you may have the same number of follicles, but thinner individual strands will make it look like there's less volume. (They're also more prone to break, and since hair growth slows as you age, the damage becomes more obvious.)

Even if you do see extra hairs in your brush or in the shower drain, you don't necessarily need to worry. Although 40 percent of women experience some hair loss by menopause, shedding around 100 strands a day is normal, reports Paul M. Friedman, M.D., clinical assistant professor of dermatology at the University of Texas Medical School at Houston."

So it may be my CKD that's causing the hair thinning or it may not. Either way, I wanted to know what to do about it. Dr. Doris Day (I kid you not.) has other suggestions than protein as she discusses in a New York Times article.

"Dr. Doris Day, a dermatologist in New York, agreed that the right foods are necessary for healthy hair.

'I believe that inflammation is negative for the hair folli-cle, that it can accelerate stress shedding and compro-mise growth,' she said. She suggests eating pomegran-ate, avocado, pumpkin and olive oil, and herbs like tur-meric, mint and rosemary."

You do remember that CKD is an inflammatory disease, right? Hmmm, better check with your renal nutritionist before you start eating pomegranates or pumpkin. They're on my NO! list, but yours may be different from mine.

By the way, I've noticed there are no reviews for *SlowItDownCKD 2015* on either Amazon.com or B&N.com. Can you help a writer out here? Just click on either site name to leave a review. Thanks.

8/1/16 *Maybe for You, But Not for Me*

Last week, when I wrote about thinning hair, I received loads of suggestions. While I was pleased with all the interaction, it was clear to me that we had people answering from three different positions: pre-dialysis (like me at Stage 3 Chronic Kidney Disease), dialysis, and post-transplant. What also became clear is that the 'rules' for each position are different. That got me to wondering.

But first, I think a definition of each of these is necessary. My years teaching English ingrained in me that 'pre' is a prefix meaning before; so pre-dialysis means before dialysis. In other words, this is CKD stages 1-4 or 5 depending upon your nephrologist. It's when there is a slow progression in the decline of your kidney function.

I remembered a definition of dialysis that I liked in *SlowItDownCKD 2015*, and so, decided to repeat it here.

"According to the National Kidney Foundation,

'Dialysis is a treatment that does some of the things done by healthy kidneys. It is needed when your own kidneys can no longer take care of your body's needs. There are several different kinds of dialysis. Basically, they each eliminate the wastes and extra fluid in your blood via different methods.'"

And post -transplant? Simply put, it means after having had a kidney (or other organ) placed in your body to replace one that doesn't work anymore.

I know as a pre-dialysis that I have certain dietary re-strictions. Readers have told me some of theirs and they're very different. It's not the usual difference based on lab results that will tell you whether you need to cut back more on one of the electrolytes this quarter. It seemed like an entirely different system.

Let's go back to *What Is It and How Did I Get It? Early Stage Chronic Kidney Disease* to see what my basic die-tary restrictions as a pre-dialysis CKD patient are.

 "The (e.g. renal) diets seem to agree that protein, sodi-um, phosphorus and potassium need to be limited. … Apparently, your limits may be different from mine or any other patient's. In other words, it's personalized."

Well, what about those on dialysis? What do their die-tary guidelines look like? I found this in *The Book of Blogs: Moderate Stage Chronic Kidney Disease, Part 2*:

"Knowing End Stage Renal Disease is not my area of ex-pertise, I took a peek at National Kidney and Urologic Diseases Information Clearinghouse (NKUDIC), a service of the National Institute of Diabetes and Digestive and Kidney Diseases (NIDDK), National Institutes of Health (NIH), anyway to see what dialysis patients can eat.

'Potassium is a mineral found in many foods, especially milk, fruits, and vegetables. It affects how steadily your heart beats. Healthy kidneys keep the right amount of potassium in the blood to keep the heart beating at a steady pace. Potassium levels can rise between dialysis sessions and affect your heartbeat. Eating too much potassium can be very dangerous to your heart. It may even cause death.'"

I suspected that potassium is not the only dietary problem for dialysis and dug a bit more. I discovered this information on MedicineNet, along with the caveat that these also need to be individualized as per lab results.

1. Fluids: Allowance is based primarily on the type of dialysis and urine output. If you have any edema, are taking a diuretic, and/or have congestive heart failure, your allowance will be adjusted.

2. Sodium: This will be modified to maintain blood pressure and fluid control and to help prevent congestive heart failure and pulmonary edema.

3. Potassium: Your intake of this will be adjusted to prevent your blood levels from going too high or too low.

4. Phosphorus: The majority of dialysis patients require phosphate binders and dietary restrictions in order to control their blood phosphorus levels.

5. Protein: Adequate protein is necessary to maintain and replenish your stores. You may be instructed on increasing your intake now that you are on dialysis.

6. Fiber: There is a chance that constipation may be a problem due to fluid restrictions and phosphate binders, so it's important to keep fiber intake up. You will need guidance on this because many foods that are high in fiber are also high in potassium.

7. Fat: Depending on your blood cholesterol levels, you may need to decrease your intake of trans fat, saturated fat, and cholesterol.

8. Calories: If you are over or underweight, you will be instructed on adjusting the amount of calories that you take in each day.

9. Calcium: Most foods that contain calcium also contain phosphorus. Due to your phosphorus restrictions, you will need guidance on how to get enough calcium while limiting your intake of phosphorus.

Big difference here! More protein, less calcium, phosphate binders, fat and calcium. No wonder the responses I got to last week's blog were so varied.

And post-transplant? What about those dietary restrictions? The Mayo Clinic has that one covered, with the same warning as the other two groups' diets: your labs dictate your amounts.

- Eating at least five servings of fruits and vegetables each day

- Avoiding grapefruit and grapefruit juice due to its effect on a group of immunosuppression medications (calcineurin inhibitors)

- Having enough fiber in your daily diet

- Drinking low-fat milk or eating other low-fat dairy products, which is important to maintain optimal calcium and phosphorus levels

- Eating lean meats, poultry and fish

- Maintaining a low-salt and low-fat diet

- Following food safety guidelines

- Staying hydrated by drinking adequate water and other fluids each day

So it looks like you get to eat more servings of fruits and vegetables a day, must avoid grapefruit and its juice, and be super vigilant about calcium and phosphorus levels. Notice the same suggestion to have enough fiber in your diet as when on dialysis.

Whoa! We have three different sets of diet guidelines for three different stages of CKD, along with the strict understanding that everything depends upon your lab results. That means that the post-transplant patients were right – for them – that I needed more pro-tein. And the dialysis patients were right – for them – too. But for the pre-dialysis patients? Nope, got to stay below five ounces daily.

8/8/16 *CKD Treatment Interruptus*

Recently, someone close to me experienced a major burglary. After calling the police, he called me. That's what my friends do and I'm thankful they do. I kept him on the phone while I threw on some clothes and sped over to his house. This is a strong, independent man who was shocked at the intimacy of the invasion of his home. When I got there, we walked from room to room, astonished at how much had been stolen.

That night, I couldn't leave – not even to go home for my evening medications and supplements. That night, I couldn't sleep while my buddy was in such turmoil. So we sat up staring at the empty space where the TV had been. He's not on the renal diet and all he had that I could eat was some chicken, no fruit, no vegetables. And I was too busy being with him to exercise. This was my good buddy of over 30 years standing.

The next morning, another friend came over to help with security devices and spend time with our mutual friend. I got to go home, take my morning medications, and crawl into bed for ½ an hour. But then our mutual friend had to go to work, so I went back to my buddy's house and spent the day helping him try to list what was missing, what to do about the insurance, how to handle going to work, etc. The word spread, and, suddenly, a third friend was coming to spend the night with him and another couple joined them to make dinner. I could go home again.

But I was exhausted. I ate stupidly: Chinese restaurant food with all that sodium. I even ate rice, and here I am on a low carbohydrate diet. I sat in the living room like a zombie while Bear waited on me hand and foot.

Even with all this help, my buddy needed to see me daily. I was his strength. So we ran around rummaging up some receipts he'd need for the insurance. But I could see he was feeling better. Our mutual friends were amazing, including those who couldn't leave work to come so kept phoning and texting instead. A different someone else stayed with him overnight again. Then he only needed to see me for a quick hug... and yet another someone else stayed with him overnight again. He didn't really need me anymore, which is great because I started breaking down.

I have Chronic Kidney Disease. I need to sleep adequately – and with my BiPAP. I need to follow the renal diet. I need to exercise. I need to rest. I did very little of any of this during the trauma itself, and that's alright. This is my long term buddy – as grown up and mature as he is – and he needed me. But what did I do to myself?

You guessed it. Right away, my blood pressure shot up and that's a bad thing. Why? Let me tell you... or you can go to *What Is It and How Did I Get It? Early Stage Chronic Kidney Disease*, page 9.

"Through my research, I began to understand what high blood pressure [**HPB**] has to do with renal disease. HPB can damage small blood vessels in the kidneys to the point that they cannot filter the waste from the blood as effectively as they should. Nephrologists may prescribe HBP medication to prevent your CKD from getting worse since these medications reduce the amount of protein in your urine. Not too surprisingly, most CKD related deaths are caused by cardiovascular problems."

What about the stress? What was that doing to my poor overworked kidneys? I went to *The Book of Blogs: Moderate Stage Chronic Kidney Disease, Part 2* for the answer to that one:

"First you feel the fight or flight syndrome which means you are releasing hormones. The adrenal glands which secrete these hormones lay right on top of your kidneys. Your blood sugar raises, too, and there's an increase in both heart rate and blood pressure. Diabetes {Blood sugar} and hypertension {Blood pressure} both play a part in Chronic Kidney Disease."

That's two strikes against me. I almost hesitate to think about exercise… or the lack of it for several consecutive days. This is one of the points about treating prediabetes (which I have and so do so many of you) from the Mayo Clinic which was included in *SlowItDownCKD 2015:*

"Losing excess pounds. If you're overweight, losing just 5 to 10 percent of your body weight — only 10 to 20 pounds (4.5 to 9 kilograms) if you weigh 200 pounds (91 kilograms) — can reduce the risk of developing type 2 diabetes. To keep your weight in a healthy range, focus on permanent changes to your eating and exercise habits. Motivate yourself by remembering the benefits of losing weight, such as a healthier heart, more energy and improved self-esteem."

And the renal diet? We mustn't forget about the renal diet. In *The Book of Blogs: Moderate Kidney Disease, Part 1* I quoted Yourkidneys.com from DaVita:

"Depending on what stage of Chronic Kidney Disease you're in, your renal dietitian will adjust the amounts of protein, sodium, phosphorus and potassium in your diet. In addition, carbohydrates and fats may be controlled based on conditions such as diabetes and cardiovascular disease. The CKD non-dialysis diet includes calculated amounts of high quality protein. Damaged kidneys have a difficult time getting rid of protein waste products, so cutting back on non-essential protein will put less stress on your kidneys."

Have I done more permanent damage to my kidneys? I'm hoping not since it was just a few days and I made the conscious decision to be with my buddy instead of tending to myself. Let's consider this a cautionary tale instead.

8/15/16 *Teachers Teach*

Many of you have asked that I post the interview by The American Federation of Teachers. I aim to please, so here it is.

From NYC teacher to international health advocate

Posted August 9, 2016 by Liza Frenette

Gail Rae-Garwood talks and writes all the time about slowing down — but she's not referring to her lifestyle speed. She's talking about putting the brakes on Chronic Kidney Disease.

When this retired high school English teacher and United Federation of Teachers member was diagnosed with CKD in 2008, she was shocked. A new doctor detected unhealthy levels for kidney functioning in routine blood and urine workups. She was sent to a nephrologist. "I didn't know what it was and what it meant," she said. "I was terrified and thought I had nowhere to turn."

She began researching and finding ways to manage this inflammatory disease through a specialized, calibrated diet, exercise, stress reduction and proper sleep. Then she realized she wanted to help others steer toward solutions. Rae-Garwood writes a weekly blog, a daily post and has published four books designed for people with CKD. She answers questions from around the world. She has spoken at coffee shops, Kiwanis Clubs, independent bookstores and senior citizen centers.

She's been a guest blogger for the American Kidney Fund, which promotes prevention activities and educational resources, and provides financial assistance for clinical research and for kidney patients who need help with dialysis and transplants.

While she is careful about getting enough sleep and eating right, Rae-Garwood does not let any waking time slip by unnoticed. She has been interviewed on Online with Andrea, The Edge Podcast, Working with Chronic Illness, and Improve Your Kidney Help. She has been interviewed for the *Wall Street Journal's* Health Matters and The Center for Science in The Public Interest.

Her action is not all talk. She also puts on the sneakers: In addition to her regular walks for health, she hustled up a team for the National Kidney Foundation of Arizona Kidney Walk.

By now, even her heart is probably kidney shaped.

Rae-Garwood also organized several talks at the Salt River Pima-Maricopa Indian Community, not far from where she lives in Arizona.

Blacks, Hispanics, Native Americans and Asians are more prone to CKD, she said. "I wanted to bring awareness everywhere I could."

Education is vital because so many people are unaware they even have the disease. Rae-Garwood is one of many who did not have any symptoms. "Many, like me, never experienced any noticeable symptoms. Many, like me, may have had high blood pressure (hypertension) for years before (CKD) was diagnosed. Yet, high blood pressure and diabetes are the two leading causes of CKD."

And CKD, left unchecked and untreated, can wreak havoc and death. According to the American Association of Kidney Patients, "The increase of kidney disease is now reaching epidemic proportions. The rates are even higher among racial and ethnic minorities. Chronic kidney disease can progress to end-stage renal disease and the need for dialysis or a kidney transplant."

Rae-Garwood's goal is to educate people and help them with their health. "You can slow down the progress of the decline of kidney function," she said.

And she is the very living proof that people want to see.

"I have been spending a lot of time on my health and I'm happy to say it's been paying off. There are five stages. I've stayed at the middle one for nine years and even improved my health. That's what this is about. People don't know about CKD. They get diagnosed. They think they're going to die. Everybody dies, but it doesn't have to be of CKD. I am downright passionate about people knowing this," she said.

After her first book was published, Rae-Garwood received an e-mail from a doctor in India. He said his patients were extremely poor and could not afford the book – yet the information she wrote about was so important to them.

"He asked how I could help. I thought: 'I could write a blog!'" she said. Her efforts began by putting her book chapters on the blog, piece by piece. The doctor in India printed them and gave them to his patients. Newer blog posts have more up-to-date information, keeping patients informed.

Her informational blog has 106,000 readers from 107 different countries, she said, based on a report from WordPress. On her blog, Rae-Garwood answers questions from readers, lists books about CKD, reports on events, lists support groups, etc. She writes about things that have worked for her, such as using a stationary bike and stretching bands, and walking — and cautions readers to seek advice from their doctor.

The year-round outdoor climate in Arizona helps Rae-Garwood stay active. While she loved living on Staten Island, she said she owned an old Victorian that she could not afford to fix up in retirement. With an arthritis condition, she also noticed that she was "becoming a bit of a shut-in in the winter." So she moved to the southwest two months after retiring.

Rae-Garwood is not letting any of that sunshine go to waste. Since her 2008 diagnosis, she's been driving on a steady road to wellness and spreading awareness like a modern day Johnny Appleseed. In her retirement from teaching, she has devoted much time to writing, speaking and teaching about how to thwart the disease. The skills she developed in 32 years as a teacher in Brooklyn, Staten Island, Queens and Manhattan have served her well in this new role as health advocate.

Her own four self-published books are *"SlowItDownCKD 2015," "The Book of Blogs, Moderate Stage Kidney Disease Part 1," "The Book of Blogs, Moderate Stage Kidney Disease Part 2"* **and** *"What Is It and How Did I Get It? Early Stage Chronic Kidney Disease."* The books are available online at Barnes and Noble and Amazon.

For more information on the disease and this active, 69-year-old retiree, check out *https://gailraegarwood.wordpress.com*.

I hope that this interview has been both enjoyable and informative. It's how I live my life...

8/22/16 *Not Quite the Bionic Woman*

I have a knee brace. The little sucker goes from mid-calf to mid-thigh... and it's going to have a twin for the other knee. I'm sort of disappointed because I thought it was going to be solely for when I exercise daily. Only that's not true; it's going to be for eight hours a day. How did I so misunderstand what the doctor was saying?

More importantly, what the heck is this for? I double checked this with the rheumatologist: it's to postpone knee surgery as long as possible. As I understand it, there's even a possibility of avoiding the surgery all to-gether. I like that option. It's also meant to minimize the pain. I like that, too.

The culprit here is osteoarthritis, which has worsened with age. Lucky me. All those years of dance, judo, Tai Chi, Aikido, and stage movement have done a job on my knees. That doesn't mean I stop dancing or exercising, though. It also doesn't mean I start taking more medica-tions, either. Hey! I have Chronic Kidney Disease.

Let's do our usual back tracking here. First question: What is osteoarthrosis of the knee? The American Academy of Orthopaedic Surgeons has a wonderfully clear explanation:

"Osteoarthritis is the most common form of arthritis in the knee. It is a degenerative, 'wear-and-tear' type of arthritis that occurs most often in people 50 years of age and older, but may occur in younger people, too. In

161

osteoarthritis, the cartilage in the knee joint gradually wears away. As the cartilage wears away, it becomes frayed and rough, and the protective space between the bones decreases. This can result in bone rubbing on bone, and produce painful bone spurs. Osteoarthritis develops slowly and the pain it causes worsens over time."

Well, that explains why the knees clicking isn't a source of amusement anymore and why getting on my knees to play with sweet Ms. Bella is now agony.

As for medications, sure NSAIDS will help... except I can't take them. Here's a reminder why not from *What Is It and How Did I Get It? Early Stage Chronic Kidney Disease*:

 "**NSAID**: Non-steroidal anti-inflammatory drugs such as ibuprofen, aspirin, Aleve or naproxen usually used for arthritis or pain management, can worsen kidney disease, sometimes irreversibly."

I'll pass on those. I do take Limbrel, though. That's not a NSAID and does help with the pain of arthritis. In *The Book of Blogs: Moderate Stage Chronic Kidney Disease, Part 1*, I defined Limbrel:

"a food medication {By prescription only} to deal with the pain preventatively."

So now we understand why the knee braces (and the Limbrel). They – the braces – supposedly fit under your clothes. Uh, no, not if you're a woman who wants to wear anything remotely stylish or not live in longish skirts. I could not get my capris or slacks on over the brace. Living in Arizona, longish skirts may work in the winter time, but they are too damned hot for the summer... which lasts from early May to late October.

So, how do these babies work you ask. I went over to the manufacturer's website for the answer to that one.

"The Unloader One applies a gentle force design to reduce the pressure on the affected part of the knee, resulting in reduction in pain and thus allowing the patient to use the knee normally and more frequently.

Untreated, the cartilage will gradually wear down. The increased pressure on the underlying bone is the cause of the pain experienced by most osteoarthritis (OA) sufferers. The wear and tear on the cartilage will gradually cause the knee to become painful and feel stiff when moving."

I wanted to know a bit more about how the knee works. The National Institute of Health explained in detail.

Bones and Cartilage

The knee joint is the junction of three bones: the femur (thigh bone or upper leg bone), the tibia (shin bone or larger bone of the lower leg), and the patella (kneecap). ...The ends of the three bones in the knee joint are covered with articular cartilage, a tough, elastic material that helps absorb shock and allows the knee joint to move smoothly. Separating the bones of the knee are pads of connective tissue called menisci (men-NISS-sky). ...The two menisci in each knee act as shock absorbers, cushioning the lower part of the leg from the weight of the rest of the body as well as enhancing stability.

Muscles

There are two groups of muscles at the knee. The four quadriceps muscles on the front of the thigh work to straighten the knee from a bent position. The hamstring muscles, which run along the back of the thigh from the hip to just below the knee, help to bend the knee.

Tendons and Ligaments

The quadriceps tendon connects the quadriceps muscle to the patella and provides the power to straighten the knee. The following four ligaments connect the femur and tibia and give the joint strength and stability:

- The medial collateral ligament, which runs along the inside of the knee joint, provides stability to the inner (medial) part of the knee.

- The lateral collateral ligament, which runs along the outside of the knee joint, provides stability to the outer (lateral) part of the knee.

- The anterior cruciate ligament, in the center of the knee, limits rotation and the forward movement of the tibia.

- The posterior cruciate ligament, also in the center of the knee, limits backward movement of the tibia.

The knee capsule is a protective, fiber-like structure that wraps around the knee joint. Inside the capsule, the joint is lined with a thin, soft tissue called synovium."

CKD brings a new way of thinking about every part of your body... even your knees. Think about it.

8/30/16 *The Nutrition Action Health Letter Article*

I am now officially excited. I'd been getting some comments about this article which I thought wasn't being published until September. I wondered why. It was my mistake. The article was to appear in the September issue, which I didn't realize is published before the month begins.

The Center for Science in the Public Interest's *September Nutrition Action Health Letter* is out. Many thanks to Bonnie Liebman for such a fine job of reporting and aiding in spreading Chronic Kidney Disease Awareness. It's long, six pages, so what we have here are excerpts.

"I didn't know that I had end-stage renal disease until I was admitted to the hospital in 2009," says David White, who was then in his mid-40s. "A few days later, I stopped producing urine."

Doctors told White that he had crashed. "It was scary," he says. "I went from 'Something may be wrong' to 'Oh my god am I going to die?' to 'I have to spend the rest of my life on dialysis.'"

And with four hours of dialysis three times a week, he never felt great.

"People call it the dialysis hangover," says White, from Temple Hills, Maryland. "You're so tired that you want to sleep all day after dialysis and most of the following day. And then you gear up for the next treatment."

And White struggled with his one-quart-a-day limit on fluids. "When you drink too much, moving isn't comfortable, laying down isn't comfortable," he says. "It's hard to breathe."

For Gail Rae-Garwood, the news about her kidneys came when she switched to a new doctor closer to her home in Glendale, Arizona.

"She decided that as a new patient, I should have all new tests," says Rae-Garwood, now 69. "When the results came in, she got me an appointment with a nephrologist the next day. When you get an appointment with a specialist the next day, you know something is not right."

Rae-Garwood had chronic kidney disease. "My GFR was down to 39, and apparently had been low for quite a while," she says. (Your GFR, or glomerular filtration rate, is the rate at which your kidneys filter your blood.) "'What is chronic kidney disease and how did I get it?' I demanded," recalls Rae-Garwood.

Every 30 minutes, your kidneys filter all the blood in your body. Without at least one, you need dialysis or a transplant. Yet most people have no idea how well their kidneys are working. "It's very common for people to have no idea that they have early chronic kidney disease," says Alex Chang, a nephrologist at Geisinger Health System in Danville, Pennsylvania.

A routine blood test sent to a major lab—like Quest or LabCorp—typically includes your GFR. If it doesn't, your doctor can calculate it.

"A GFR is pretty routine for anyone who has blood work done," says Chang. "But if you have very mild kidney disease, and especially if you're older, a doctor might not mention it since kidney function tends to decline as you age."

Doctors also look for kidney disease by testing your urine for a protein called albumin …. "That's usually only done if you have high blood pressure or diabetes or some risk factor for kidney disease other than age," says Chang.

Rae-Garwood's previous doctor missed that memo. "I had been on medication for high blood pressure for decades," she explains. "I wonder how much more of my kidney function I could have preserved if I'd known about it earlier."

***

David White had kidney transplant in 2015. "It's given me my life back," he says. "No more dialysis."

He takes anti-rejection drugs and steroids, and, like Rae-Garwood, he gets exercise and has to watch what he eats.

"I've changed my diet radically," says Rae-Garwood. "I have to limit the three P's—protein, potassium, and phosphorus. I'm restricted to 5 ounces of protein a day. We have no red meat in the house. Any product above 7 or 8 percent of a day's worth of sodium I don't buy.

"And you know what? It's fine. It's been nine years now, and I've been able to keep my GFR around 50."

Both patients are now advocates for preventing kidney disease. "I've written four books and almost 400 weekly blogs, and I post a daily fact about chronic kidney disease on Facebook," says Rae-Garwood. White chairs the MidAtlantic Renal Coalition's patient advisory committee, among other things among other things.

"Get tested," urges Rae-Garwood. "Millions of people have chronic kidney disease and don't even know it. All it takes is a blood and urine test."

My hope is that as a result of this article, more libraries, medical schools, and nephrology practices will order copies of *What Is It and How Did I Get It? Early Stage Chronic Kidney Disease*, *The Book of Blogs: Moderate Stage Chronic Kidney Disease, Part 1*, *The Book of Blogs: Moderate Stage Chronic Kidney Disease, Part 2*, and *SlowItDownCKD 2015*. If you have a Kindle, Amazon has two wonderful low cost or free programs that may make it easier for you, your loved ones, and anyone you think could benefit from these books to read them.

This is how Amazon explains these programs:

"Kindle Unlimited is a subscription program for readers that allows them to read as many books as they want. The Kindle Owners' Lending Library is a collection of books that Amazon Prime members who own a Kindle can choose one book from each month with no due dates."

Barnes and Noble doesn't have any such programs, but they do offer discount deals daily, which you can use to purchase any book.

I urge you to help spread awareness of Chronic Kidney Disease in any way you can. Here's another quote from the article that may help you understand why:

"One out of ten adults has chronic kidney disease. Most don't know it because early on, kidney disease has no symptoms. And because the risk rises as you age, roughly one out of two people aged 30 to 64 are likely to get the disease during their lives...."

9/5/16 *Feeling the Pressure*

For those of you in the United States, here's hoping you have a healthy, safe Labor Day. I come from a Union family. So much so that my maternal grandfather was in and out of jail for attempting to unionize brass workers. That was quite a bit of pressure on my grandmother, who raised the four children and ran a restaurant.

I knew there was more than my personal history with the holiday so I poked around and found this from USA Today.

"In the late 1800s, the state of labor was grim as U.S. workers toiled under bleak conditions: 12 or more hour workdays; hazardous work environments; meager pay. Children, some as young as 5, were often fixtures at plants and factories.

The dismal livelihoods fueled the formation of the country's first labor unions, which began to organize strikes and protests and pushed employers for better hours and pay. Many of the rallies turned violent.

On Sept. 5, 1882 — a Tuesday — 10,000 workers took unpaid time off to march in a parade from City Hall to Union Square in New York City as a tribute to American workers. Organized by New York's Central Labor Union, It was the country's first unofficial Labor Day parade. Three years later, some city ordinances marked the first government recognition, and legislation soon followed in a number of states."

Now that's pressure, but I want to write about another kind of pressure today: your blood pressure.

Being one of those people who is required to check their blood pressure at least once a day, I was surprised to learn that doctors didn't realize the importance of maintaining moderate blood pressure until the 1950s. Yet, ancient Chinese, Greeks, and Egyptians knew about the pulse. I wonder what they thought that was.

The American Heart Association explains the difference between the blood pressure and the pulse, and offers a chart to exemplify. The column without the heading refers to '**Heart Rate.**'

	Blood Pressure	
What is it?	The force the heart exerts against the walls of arteries as it pumps the blood out to the body	The number of times your heart beats per minute
What is the unit of measure-ment?	mm Hg (millimeters of mercury)	BPMs (beats per minute)
What do the numbers repre-sent?	Includes two meas-urements: **Systolic pressure (top number):** The	Includes a sin-gle number representing the number of

	Blood Pressure	
	pressure as the heart beats and forces blood into the arteries **Diastolic pressure (bottom num- ber):** The pressure as the heart relaxes between beats	heart beats per minute
Sample reading	120/80 mm Hg	60 BPM

According to Withings, a French company that sells blood pressure monitoring equipment:

"The first study on blood circulation was published in 1628 by William Harvey – an English physician. He came to the conclusion that the heart acts as a pump. At that point it wasn't clear that blood circulated, but after a little calculation he was pretty sure that blood is not 'consumed' by the organs. The physician then conclud- ed that blood must be going though (sic) a cycle."

Ah, but did his measurement include both numbers? In *What Is It and How Did I Get It? Early Stage Chronic Kidney Disease*, I satisfied my own curiosity as to why our blood pressure readings always have two numbers, one atop the other:

"The first number... called the systolic is the rate at which the heart contracts, while the second or diastolic ... is when the heart is at rest between contractions. These numbers measure the units of millimeters of mercury to which your heart has raised the mercy."

Uh, raised the mercury of what? Well it's not the sphygmomanometer as we now know it. By the way, this is the connection between blood pressure and Chronic Kidney Disease that I mentioned in *SlowItDownCKD 2015*:

"I wonder how frustrated Dr. Bright became when he first suspected that hypertension had a strong effect on the kidneys, but had no way to prove that theory since the first practical sphygmomanometer (Me here: That's the device that measures your blood pressure.) wasn't yet available."

Well, why is hypertension – high blood pressure – important in taking care of your kidneys anyway? It's the second leading cause of CKD. The Mayo Clinic succinctly explains why -

"Your kidneys filter excess fluid and waste from your blood — a process that depends on healthy blood vessels. High blood pressure can injure both the blood vessels in and leading to your kidneys, causing several types of kidney disease (nephropathy). "

Well, how do you avoid it then? One way is to take the pressure off yourself. (As a writer, I'm thoroughly enjoying that this kind of pressure can affect the other kind – the blood pressure. As a CKD patient, I'm not.)

Pressure on yourself is usually considered stress. In *The Book of Blogs: Moderate Stage Chronic Kidney Disease, Part 2*, there's an explanation of what stress does to your body.

"...we respond the same way whether the stress is positive or negative.... First you feel the fight or flight syndrome which means you are releasing hormones. The adrenal glands which secrete these hormones lay right on top of your kidneys. Your blood sugar raises, too, and there's an increase in both heart rate and blood pressure. Diabetes {High blood sugar} and hypertension {High blood pressure} both play a part in Chronic Kidney Disease. If you still haven't resolved the stress, additional hormones are secreted for more energy."

What else? This list from the American Kidney Fund was included in *The Book of Blogs: Moderate Stage Chronic Kidney Disease, Part 1:*

- Eat a diet low in salt and fat

- Be physically active

- Keep a healthy weight

- Control your cholesterol

- Take medicines as directed

- Limit alcohol

- Avoid tobacco

Why am I not surprised at how much this looks like the list for healthy kidneys?

I was just thinking: what better day to start working on this list than Labor Day?

9/12/16 *The Lamp Post and the Kidneys*

This past week, my car and I tangled with a lamp post. My car got the worst of it. Luckily, I was driving very slowly in a parking lot while looking for the Disabled Parking Spots. (Ironic, isn't it?) All I got were bruises and stiffness. Or did I?

As usual when confronted with something I didn't know about, I started wondering: What happened to my kidneys safely buried in my body while my skin turned black and blue from the seat belt and my hand ended up with tendonitis from gripping the steering wheel so firmly?

The kidneys are internal organs, which means they are not directly under the skin, but protected by layers of fat and muscle (Hmmmm, I usually wish there were more muscle and less fat over them), and other organs.

According to The University of Michigan Medical School's Dissector Answers:

"Besides their peritoneal covering, each is embedded in two layers of fat, with a membrane, the renal fascia, in between the layers. Inside the renal fascia is the perirenal fat, while outside the membrane is the pararenal fat. (The perirenal layer is inside, while the pararenal layer is around the renal fascia.)"

Great! All I needed to know now is what that meant. We already know from the quote above that perirenal fat is inside the renal fascia, while pararenal fat is outside, but what's the fascia?

The Medical Dictionary section of the Free Dictionary cleared that up right away:

"a sheet or band of fibrous tissue such as lies deep to the skin or invests muscles and various body organs."

Wait a minute; what about peritoneal? I had this vague memory of hearing the word before, but not its definition. Just to mix it up a little bit, this time I turned to MedicineNet, but for the root word *peritoneum* since the suffix 'al' just means relating to and will only confuse the issue. ...

"The membrane that lines the abdominal cavity and covers most of the abdominal organs."

I needed the information on AnatomyZone to find out what lies in front of the kidneys.

"... the colon runs in front of the kidney. .... It runs in front of the lower part of the kidney, the inferior pole of the kidney. That's the hepatic flexure..... the descending part of the duodenum sits in front of the medial part of the kidney. The descending part of the duodenum is retroperitoneal as well and it sits right up against the kidney....on top of the kidney. This is the suprarenal gland or the adrenal gland.

.... the other side of the colon sits in front of the left kidney.... the stomach and the spleen sitting in front of it. ... the end of the pancreas sitting in front of it as well."

This reads a bit choppy because it is describing an interactive visualization of the kidneys. I found this even more entertaining than my *Concise Encyclopedia of the Human Body* (London: Red Lemon Press, 2015) which I can pore over for hours just marveling at this body of ours.

It seems to me that I've ignored whatever is behind the kidneys so let's find out what's there. Oh, of course...

"The ribs and muscles of the back protect the kidneys from external damage. Adipose tissue known as perirenal fat surrounds the kidneys and acts as protective padding." Many thanks to another interactive site, Inner Body for this information.

By the way, adipose tissue – or perirenal fat – is an energy storing fat. While necessary, too much of this makes us appear fat and can compromise our health. This is the white, belly fat mentioned in conjunction with kidney disease in *The Book of Blogs: Moderate Stage Chronic Kidney Disease, Part 2:*

"Other studies have suggested that once diagnosed with kidney disease, weight loss may slow kidney disease progression, but this is the first research study to support losing belly fat and limiting phosphorus con-

179

sumption as a possible way to prevent kidney disease from developing. Dr. Joseph Vassalotti, chief medical officer at the National Kidney Foundation 11/3/13"

It seems I've developed a sort of pattern here. We've looked in front of the kidneys and behind them. What's above them, I was beginning to wonder. Then I realized I already knew… and so do you if you've been reading my work: They lie below the diaphragm and the right is lower than the left because the liver is on the right side above the kidneys. The adrenal glands which were mentioned above are also on top of your kidneys. According to Reference.com, a new site for me:

"Adrenal glands are triangular-shaped, measure approximately 1.5 inches high and 3 inches long and are composed of two parts, according to Johns Hopkins Medicine. The outer part is the adrenal cortex, which creates cortisol, aldosterone and androgen hormones. The second part is the adrenal medulla, which creates noradrenaline and adrenaline.

Cortisol is a hormone that controls metabolism and helps the body react to stress, according to Endocrineweb. It affects the immune system and lowers inflammatory responses in the body. Aldosterone helps regulate sodium and potassium levels, blood volume and blood pressure. Androgen hormones are steroid hormones that are converted to female or male hormones in other parts of the body.

Noradrenaline helps regulate blood pressure, increasing it during times of stress, notes Endocrineweb. Adrenaline is often associated with the adrenal glands, and it increases the heart rate and blood flow to the muscles and the brain."

It looks like my kidneys and I had nothing to worry about. They're well protected from the impact of the accident. *sigh* If only my car had been as well protected...

9/19/16 *How Sweet She Is*

For 12 years, sweet Ms. Bella has positioned herself just inside my office door as I wrote, researched, edited, and formatted. For 12 years, sweet Ms. Bella has greeted me as effusively when I returned from a trip to the mailbox as she did when I returned from a trip to Alaska. For 12 years, sweet Ms. Bella has shared one sided conversations with me about any and everything. For 12 years, sweet Ms. Bella has adored me as no other being on earth ever has.

I'll miss that. Sweet Ms. Bella crossed what I'm told is called The Rainbow Bridge this morning. .. and it was my decision. I've known for months that she had lymphedema. First we tried this. Then we tried that. And finally there was nothing else left to try. I am oh-so-sad without my boon companion, but it was time. She knew it and I knew it. May your soul come back to me, my sweet Ms. Bella.

I've been sad for a while knowing that I would have to make this decision and wondering how I would know when she'd had enough. I watched...and watched...and watched, yet she made it perfectly clear when her legs wouldn't hold her up anymore and her cancerous lymph nodes started to impede her eating. She is at rest now.

What have I done to my kidneys with all this sadness, I wondered. I don't know via my lab reports because I was just tested last Thursday and didn't know about sweet Ms. Bella's cancer when my blood and urine were tested three months ago. So I did what I could to find out: I researched.

I found this on the National Kidney Foundation's site .

"**New York, NY (July 1, 2012)** – People with kidney disease who have symptoms of depression may be on the fast track to dialysis, hospitalization or death, according to a new study published in the July issue of the American Journal of Kidney Diseases, the official journal of the National Kidney Foundation."

But I'm not depressed; I'm sad. Well, what's the difference? I turned to my old buddy WebMD for some help here:

"….Also known as clinical depression, major depressive disorder, or unipolar depression, major depression is a medical condition that goes beyond life's ordinary ups and downs. Almost 18.8 million American adults experience depression each year, and women are nearly twice as likely as men to develop major depression. People with depression cannot simply 'pull themselves together' and get better. Treatment with counseling, medication, or both is key to recovery."

Since I'm one of those people who always manage to get myself back together – and fairly quickly – I'd say I'm not depressed. I do suggest you read more about depression if this strikes a chord with you.

So let's go back to sadness and the kidneys. This is from a 5/21/14 article on a site that's new to me: Medical Daily:

"'It's called heartbreak for a reason. When you're experiencing deep grief or sadness, it takes a toll on your health, too. One study from St. George's University of London found that it is actually possible to die of a broken heart — bereavement increases your risk of a heart attack or stroke by nearly double after a partner's death, the researchers discovered. We often use the term a 'broken heart' to signify the pain of losing a loved one and our study shows that bereavement can have a direct effect on the health of the heart,' Dr. Sunil Shah, senior lecturer in public health at St. George's, said in a press release .'"

There's a firm connection between heart health and kidney health. This is from *SlowItDownCKD 2015*:

"We're used to reading about anemia and high blood pressure as the connection between CKD and Heart Disease, but here are two other causes.

DaVita once again jumps in to educate us:

'High homocysteine levels: Damaged kidneys cannot remove extra homocysteine, an amino acid in the blood. High levels of homocysteine can lead to coronary artery disease, stroke and heart attack.

Calcium-phosphate levels: Damaged kidneys cannot keep calcium and phosphorus levels in balance. Often, there's too much phosphorus and calcium in the blood. When this happens, there's a risk for coronary artery disease.'"

Hmmm, just by having Chronic Kidney Disease, we run the risk of heart problems. Now sadness – maybe 'deep grief' is a more apt description – may add to that risk. As much as I love sweet Ms. Bella and will miss her, I can't honestly say this is true for me. It feels like there's a big difference between deep grief and sadness.

Just to make certain the difference between depression and sadness is clear, I'm repeating this information from *The Book of Blogs: Moderate Stage Chronic Kidney Disease, Part 2*:

"Make The Connection, a veterans' support site tells us

'Not everyone with depression has the same symptoms or feels the same way. One person might have difficulty sitting still, while another may find it hard to get out of bed each day. Other symptoms that may be signs of depression or may go along with being depressed include:

- Feeling sad or hopeless

- Losing interest in or not getting pleasure from most of your daily activities

- Gaining or losing weight

- Eating more or less than usual almost every day

- Sleeping too much or not enough almost every day

- Feeling restless and unable to sit still

- Feeling that moving takes great effort

- Feeling tired or as if you have no energy almost every day

- Feeling unworthy or guilty nearly every day

- Having low self-esteem or feeling down on yourself

- Finding it hard to focus, remember things, or make decisions nearly every day

- Feeling anxious, worried, or nervous

- Drinking more alcohol or caffeine

- Taking more of a prescription or over-the-medication than as directed

- Smoking or using tobacco more often'"

It doesn't look like my short term sadness is worsening my kidneys in any way, but if you're not sure whether you need help with yours, or if it is truly depression, seek help. It can't hurt to be careful.

9/26/16 *Not Your New Age Crystals*

Sometimes, a reader will ask a question and I'll research the answer for him/her, always explaining first that I'm not a doctor, don't claim to be one, and (s)he will need to check whatever information I offer with his/her nephrologist before acting on it. There was just such a comment this week: "Just wondering if you have any advice on Gout and its effect on Kidney disease? Mary." Advice? No. Research? Yes.

Let's establish just what gout is first. This is how it's defined in *What Is It and How Did I Get It? Early Stage Chronic Kidney Disease*:

"**gout**: particularly painful form of inflammatory arthritis characterized by a build-up of urate crystals in the joints, causing pain and inflammation."

Urate crystals? MedicineNet defines these as: "... salt derived from uric acid. When the body cannot metabolize uric acid properly, urates can build up in body tissues or crystallize within the joints."

Okay, what's uric acid then? Thanks to the Merriam Webster Online Dictionary for the definition:

"**URIC ACID**: a white odorless and tasteless nearly insoluble acid $C_5H_4N_4O_3$ that is the chief nitrogenous waste present in the urine especially of lower vertebrates (as birds and reptiles), is present in small quantity in human urine, and occurs pathologically in renal calculi {A little help here: this means a concretion usually of mineral salts around organic material found especially in hollow organs or ducts} and the tophi of gout."

Whoops, looks like I missed a definition here: tophi simply means the deposit itself.

You may be wondering what that has to do with Chronic Kidney Disease. This paragraph from *The Book of Blogs: Moderate Stage Chronic Kidney Disease, Part 1* explains:

"Researching that brought me to an English article from Arthritis Research UK which cited an American study. I'm going to reproduce only one paragraph of the article here because it brought home exactly what gout with Chronic Kidney Disease can do to your body.

'The findings were presented at Kidney Week 2011 by researcher Dr Erdal Sarac. He concluded: 'This study reveals a high prevalence of gout in patients with CKD. Male sex, advanced age, CAD, hypertension, and hyper-lipidemia were significantly associated with gout among CKD patients.'"

You may need some more definitions to fully under-stand that paragraph, so I'm reproducing these from *What Is It and How Did I Get It? Early Stage Chronic Kidney Disease*:

CAD: coronary artery disease

hyperlipidemia: high cholesterol

hypertension: high blood pressure

Gout sounds bad. I'll bet you're wondering how you can help avoid gout... especially if you have CKD. Let's go back to *The Book of Blogs: Moderate Stage Chronic Kidney Disease, Part 1* for a moment.

"One disease, CKD, can be implicated for three others if you also have gout. ... I didn't know that gout is also somehow in the mix of being medically compromised. I have hyperlipidemia and hypertension and CKD. True, I'm not an older male but should I become more vigilant about any hints of gout? ....

I would have to be careful about my food and beverage intake. Oh, wait, I'm already doing that by following the renal diet. In both, you are urged to cut back on alcohol and drink more water instead. Purines are a problem, too, but then again I am limited to five ounces of protein {a purine food source} per day. Hmmm, avoiding sugar-sweetened drinks may help. Say, with CKD, I have to watch my A1C {How the body handles glucose or sugar in a three month period} so that I don't end up with diabetes. That means I'm watching all my sugar intake already. I see fructose rich fruits can be a problem. But I'm already restricted to only three servings of fruit a day! Oh, here's the biggie: lose weight. Yep, been hearing that from my nephrologist for four (Me here: it's more like nine years now.) years. To sum up, by attending to my CKD on a daily basis, I'm also at-tempting to avoid or lessen the effects of gout.

This is getting very interesting. I also take medication for both hypertension and hyperlipidemia. Are they also helping me to avoid gout? It seems to me that by treating one condition {Or two in my case}, I'm also treating my CKD and possibly preventing another. It is all inter-related."

By the way, based upon another reader's question I mentioned cherries and gout in *The Book of Blogs: Moderate Stage Chronic Kidney Disease, Part 2*:

"From my reading, I've also garnered the information that cherries can help with iron deficiencies, lower blood pressure, improve sleep, help with gout, and low-er the risk of heart disease.

Or can they? Remember that too much potassium can actually cause an irregular heartbeat or possibly stop your heart."

So now, we need to watch purines and potassium, too. Aha! Following the renal diet already is helping to avoid potassium. What about purines? According to WebMD:

"Purines (specific chemical compounds found in some foods) are broken down into uric acid. A diet rich in pu-rines from certain sources can raise uric acid levels in the body, which sometimes leads to gout. Meat and seafood may increase your risk of gout. Dairy products may lower your risk."

It seems to me a small list of high purine foods is appropriate here. Gout Education offers just that. This also appears to be an extremely helpful site for those wanting to know more about gout.

"Because uric acid is formed from the breakdown of purines, high-purine foods can trigger attacks. It is strongly encouraged to avoid:

- Beer and grain liquors

- Red meat, lamb and pork

- Organ meats, such as liver, kidneys and sweetbreads

- Seafood, especially shellfish, like shrimp, lobster, mussels, anchovies and sardines"

Does this list sound familiar? It should if you're following the renal diet. While not exactly the same, there's quite a bit of overlap in the two diets.

Mary… and every other reader… I hope this was enough information for you to write a list of questions about CKD and gout to bring to your next nephrology appointment.

10/3/16 *Then Why Wait?*

It's that time of year again, ladies and gentlemen. Time for what, you ask. Well, yes, it is almost time for Halloween (and my fellow writer brother's Halloween birthday) but it's also time for your flu shot… or jab, depending upon which part of the world you're in. I've written before about why it's important to have this protection, especially if you're getting older – like me. But I don't think I've written about why it's a good idea to wait.

"'If you're over 65, don't get the flu vaccine in September. Or August. It's a marketing scheme,' said Laura Haynes, an immunologist at the University of Connecticut Center on Aging," in the same NPR article referred to later in this blog. Considering the information my own immunologist gave me, I have to agree. But, here we are back to what my cousin calls my probing question: why?

According to the CDC (Centers for Disease Control and Prevention):

"Getting vaccinated before flu activity begins helps protect you once the flu season starts in your community. It takes about two weeks after vaccination for the body's immune response to fully respond and for you to be protected so make plans to get vaccinated. CDC recommends that people get a flu vaccine by the end of October, if possible. However, getting vaccinated later can still be beneficial. CDC recommends ongoing flu vaccination as long as influenza viruses are circulating, even into January or later."

Wait a minute. How do the private companies that produce the flu vaccine know what strains to include protection against? NPR (National Public Radio) has something to say about that:

"To develop vaccines, manufacturers and scientists study what's circulating in the Southern Hemisphere during its winter flu season — June, July and August. Then, based on that evidence, they forecast what flu strains might be circulating in the U.S. the following November, December and January, and incorporate that information into flu vaccines that are generally ready by late July."

Nope, still doesn't answer my question. I decided to turn to CNN :

"'... antibodies created by the vaccine decline in the months following vaccination 'primarily affecting persons age 65 and older,' citing a study done during the 2011-2012 flu season. Still, while 'delaying vaccination might permit greater immunity later in the season,' the CDC notes that 'deferral could result in missed opportunities to vaccinate.'"

This is in keeping with what my own immunologist and my PCP (primary care physician) both warned me. Bear is 70. I'm close to it. We won't be having our inoculations until later in October. Which brings us around to the question of why have the flu shot at all?

The England's Department of Health chart included in *The Book of Blogs: Moderate Stage Chronic Kidney Disease, Part 2* partially answers this question:

Even if you feel healthy, you should definitely consider having the free {In England, that is} seasonal flu vaccination if you have:

- a heart problem

- a chest complaint or breathing difficulties, including bronchitis or emphysema

- ***a kidney disease*** {I bolded and italicized this for obvious reasons.}

- lowered immunity due to disease or treatment (such as steroid medication or cancer treatment)

- a liver disease

- had a stroke or a transient ischaemic attack (TIA)

- diabetes

- a neurological condition, for example multiple sclerosis (MS) or cerebral palsy

- a problem with your spleen, for example sickle cell disease or you have had your spleen removed.

I found this little nugget that's more emphatic about why Chronic Kidney Disease patients need to have the vaccine in *SlowItDownCKD 2015*:

"DaVita tells us,

'Immunizations may prevent people from contracting other diseases, infections and viruses. The immune system of a person with chronic kidney disease (CKD) becomes weakened, making it difficult to fight off many diseases and infections. Patients with CKD may become more susceptible to illness and even death if they do not receive regular immunization treatment. Getting the proper immunizations is an essential part of a person's kidney care.'"

You've probably heard that there are different strains of the flu. I went to England's National Health Services site to discover what they are:

"There are three types of flu viruses. They are:

- **type A flu virus** – this is usually the more serious type. The virus is most likely to mutate into a new version that people are not resistant to. The H1N1 (swine flu) strain is a type A virus, and flu pandemics in the past were type A viruses.

- **type B flu virus** – this generally causes a less severe illness and is responsible for smaller outbreaks. It mainly affects young children.

- **type C flu virus** – this usually causes a mild illness similar to the common cold.

Most years, one or two strains of type A flu circulate as well as type B."

A new site for me, but one I suspect I'll be returning to in the future, Public Health explains how a vaccine works:

"A vaccine works by training the immune system to recognize and combat pathogens, either viruses or bacteria. To do this, certain molecules from the pathogen must be introduced into the body to trigger an immune response.

These molecules are called antigens, and they are present on all viruses and bacteria. By injecting these antigens into the body, the immune system can safely learn to recognize them as hostile invaders, produce antibodies, and remember them for the future. If the bacteria or virus reappears, the immune system will recognize the antigens immediately and attack aggressively well before the pathogen can spread and cause sickness."

I've already had something. I don't know it was, but it felt like a little bit of a preview for the flu and it was awful. When I become ill, I can be down for anywhere from three to six weeks. This time? Probably 10 days which, by the way, is the usual run for the common cold. Was it a cold? Strain C of the flu? I don't know, but you can bet it reinforced that I'll be getting that flu shot. Why go for more misery if I can help it?

10/10/16 *Is it CKD? Or Is It Arizona?*

I've written about my dismay at thinning hair. By the way, I've come to terms with that rather than trying any product other than a new shampoo. What helped me come to that decision was a date day picture. My hair looked like straw in that picture and probably had for a while, although I hadn't taken note of it.

It was dry, terribly dry. Well, I do live in Arizona. Our annual relative humidity index is about 31%. Thank you to Climatemps.com for this information.

For those of you (like me) who never thought about it before, I found the following excellent explanation of humidity at Britannica.com.

"Care must be taken to distinguish between the relative humidity of the air and its moisture content or density, known as absolute humidity. The air masses above the tropical deserts such as the Sahara and Mexican deserts contain vast quantities of moisture as invisible water vapour. Because of the high temperatures, however, relative humidities are very low."

Hmmm, Mexican deserts…high temperatures… yep, that's us. Wait a minute. My youngest and one of my step-daughters live here, too. They have beautiful, luxurious hair. My delightful neighbor is a little older than my daughters, but her hair is always healthy looking and attractive. Okay, I'm older but I also have Chronic Kidney Disease.

Let's take a look at what age can do to your hair first. (Saving the best for last, of course.) The Natural Society (I do occasionally check these sites.) tells us:

"Low level of thyroid hormone can cause hair loss because it slows the metabolic rate throughout the body, a reason that low thyroid and weight gain often go hand in hand. This slowing extends to scalp follicles, resulting in premature release of the hair shaft and root, and a delay in producing replacement hairs. Early graying is another indication of low thyroid, as is the loss of hairs from the temporal edges of the eyebrows."

Interesting, but it doesn't talk about dryness, just hair loss... and my thyroid levels have always been fine.

Let's try again. Prevention.com hit the nail on the head for me:

"But after you hit 40, the damage begins to go deeper, extending to the hair's inner cuticle, known as the endocuticle.

This type of damage is a result of the body's reduced ability to repair itself, says Nicole Rogers, MD, assistant clinical professor of dermatology at Tulane University. In your 20s and 30s, the body (including your hair) bounces back from outside damage fairly quickly. But as you hit middle age, hair breaks down more quickly and the outer cuticle is repaired at a slower rate, leaving the inner cuticle vulnerable to the same outside attacks it once was shielded from."

After you hit 40? That changed my entire outlook. At almost 70, I was actually lucky that I'd had so many years without dry hair. Amazing how information like this can reverse your thinking.

But I have CKD. Was this adding to the dry hair problem? I went to my old standby DaVita for help:

"... hair can become visibly abnormal when you develop a disease. Some people experience hair breakage or find that their hair falls out, or sometimes both."

That tickled my memory. Oh, I remember writing this in *What Is It and How Did I Get It? Early and Moderate Stage Chronic Kidney Disease*.

"... (oddly enough, my curly hair would become temporarily straight if I were incubating some illness or other)..."

All right, that helps a bit, but – as usual – I wanted to know why. Another old favorite, WebMD was helpful in a general, non-CKD, way:

"Your scalp isn't making enough moisture. Hair has no natural lubrication. It relies on oils made in the hair root to keep your hair moisturized and looking lustrous.

Sometimes, hair doesn't make enough oil, which leads to dry hair. (Likewise, roots in overdrive lead to oily and greasy hair.) As you age, your hair naturally makes less oil."

Well, it looks like age, humidity, and disease – including Chronic Kidney Disease – all have something to do with dry hair. I sort of, kind of, remembered hydrating my hair with some home remedy when I was younger and had caused some damage by skiing in the sun or playing in a chlorinated swimming pool too much. Something about mayonnaise. NaturallyCurley.com (How apt!) explains:

"Mayonnaise does contain some hair healthy ingredients like lemon juice, vinegar and soybean oil which contain fatty acids and vitamins that can boost shine and act to seal in moisture."

The method is simple:

1. Work the mayonnaise into your hair.

2. Put on a shower cap.

3. Leave it on for about half an hour.

4. Rinse out the mayonnaise.

5. Wash your hair with a gentle shampoo.

I tried this last night and am very happy with the results. Maybe – in this case – it is just that easy.

I want to remind you that each of the websites I mention will give you more information about the particular topic you're interested in.

I had a really nice surprise the other day and wanted to share it with you. A little background is necessary first. I was a high school English teacher in New York City for 34 years before I retired and moved to Arizona. As such, I joined my union – The United Federation of Teachers. Because I did, I'm also a member of the New York State United Teachers. They publish a newspaper which has a section entitled 'Kudos,' that applauds the accomplishments of their members.

As a retired teacher, I glance through the paper each time it arrives. I found a notice about my four Chronic Kidney Disease books in the Fall 2016 issue. Thank you, thank you, thank you. These are non-Chronic Kidney Disease people appreciating writings about Chronic Kidney Disease.

10/17/16 *And I Shall Dance the Night Away*

Once upon a time, there was a little girl who loved to dance. Her parents were ballroom dancers: smooth, gliding, and delightful to watch. She wanted to do that, too, but there were no ballroom lessons for little girls at that time. She took a tap lesson or two, but the school was too far away for her to walk or for her driving shy mother to drive.

Then there was nothing until her school offered dance lessons during the gym period, all kinds of dance: square, cha-cha, rhumba, mambo, salsa, waltz, foxtrot. That's when she realized her parents were her best dance teachers… and that dancing was in her blood. When she hit college, she went dancing with her buddies every chance she got.

Then she married, had a family, and only danced at weddings. It wasn't such a happy time for her. But her children grew up and she found she could take them to swing dances with her. She was happy again. One of the now adult children initiated and taught blues dance lessons every week. She was ecstatic.

That group is Sustainable Blues, Phoenix, and that child is Abby Wegerski. The little dancer grown up? It's me, as if you hadn't guessed by now. And here's comes the reason for the dancing introduction to this week's blog.

We have Chronic Kidney Disease; we need to exercise at least half an hour a day for five days a week, daily if possible. This little tidbit from *What Is It and How Did I Get It? Early Stage Chronic Kidney Disease* explains why:

"I researched, researched and researched again. Each explanation of what exercise does for the body was more complicated than the last one I read. Keeping it simple, basically, there's a compound released by voluntary muscle contraction. It tells the body to repair itself and grow stronger."

I went into this just a bit further in *The Book of Blogs: Moderate Stage Chronic Kidney Disease, Part 1*:

"With Chronic Kidney Disease, I *need* the daily exercise to keep my organs – all of them – strong, especially since CKD can eventually affect your other organs. It's our not-quite-filtered blood that feeds these organs, so we need to keep them healthy in as many ways as we can."

Okay. Got it. Now the biggie: Is dancing the exercise we think it is? I turned to WebMD for the following:

(Exercise physiologist Catherine Cram, MS, of Comprehensive Fitness Consulting in Middleton, Wis. is the one being quoted.)

"'Once someone gets to the point where they're getting their heart rate up, they're actually getting a terrific workout,' says Cram.

Dance is a weight-bearing activity, which builds bones. It's also *wonderful* for your upper body and strength, says Cram.'"

Weight-bearing? I wasn't so sure I could accept that so I turned to the National Institute of Arthritis and Musculoskeletal and Skin Diseases for verification.

"The best exercise for your bones is the weight-bearing kind, which forces you to work against gravity. Some examples of weight-bearing exercises include weight training, walking, hiking, jogging, climbing stairs, tennis, and dancing."

Look at that last word. Finally! My weight is working for me, instead of against me. Of course, I am in no way suggesting you gain weight so you can get more of the weight-bearing benefits of dancing.

But that's not the only benefit of dancing as a weight-bearing exercise. In *The Book of Blogs: Moderate Stage Chronic Kidney Disease, Part 2* I reproduced part of a Los Angeles Times article about weight-bearing exercise. Potteiger is Jeffrey Potteiger, an exercise physiologist at Grand Valley State University in Grand Rapids, Mich., and a fellow of the American College of Sports Medicine.

"Another big advantage ... is improving glucose metabolism, which can reduce the risk of diabetes. Strength training boosts the number of proteins that take glucose out of the blood and transport it into the skeletal muscle, giving the muscles more energy and lowering overall blood-glucose levels.

'If you have uncontrolled glucose levels,' Potteiger said, 'that can lead to kidney damage, damage to the circulatory system and loss of eyesight.'"

I found the following list on the website of Australia's Victoria State Government Better Health Channel and was delighted at just how much we benefit ourselves when we dance.

Health benefits of dancing

Dancing can be a way to stay fit for people of all ages, shapes and sizes. It has a wide range of physical and mental benefits including:

- improved condition of your heart and lungs

- increased muscular strength, endurance and motor fitness

- increased aerobic fitness

- improved muscle tone and strength

- weight management

- stronger bones and reduced risk of osteoporosis

- better coordination, agility and flexibility

- improved balance and spatial awareness

- increased physical confidence

- improved mental functioning

- improved general and psychological wellbeing

- greater self-confidence and self-esteem

- better social skills.

Wow - just wow. Who knew that the little girl who loved dancing would grow up to be the woman who used what she loved to keep her Chronic Kidney Disease under control?

After all this good news – actually joyful to me – I unfortunately have to end this week's blog on a cautionary note. It's been brought to my attention AGAIN that students are being tricked into wasting their money by renting my Chronic Kidney Disease books for more than it would cost to buy them or asking their libraries to order copies to be borrowed for free. So, here's the same warning I published earlier this year in *SlowItDownCKD 2015*.

"Students: do NOT rent any of these for a semester. The cost for that is much higher than buying the book. Having been a college instructor, I know you sometimes have to buy your textbooks before the class begins and the instructor has the chance to tell you this."

College has changed. It's no longer two or three terms a year. Many colleges have staggered start dates, some weekly, some monthly. Many of the duped students used their financial aid money to pay these book rental companies. Be careful, students.

10/24/16 *Updates, Anyone?*

Several months ago, an Arizona reader asked me to meet her for lunch to talk over her Chronic Kidney Disease journey and mine. I was open to the idea and glad to be able to share ideas with each other.

Uh-oh, during the conversation, while trying to share my iPhone apps with her, I discovered that one of those I use to help me is no longer available to new installers. That got me to thinking about what else may have changed in the CKD electronic world.

Time to back track just a bit. I have an iPhone and look for apps for those. Many of the apps I looked at are also available for Androids, iPads, and iPod Touch. According to GCFLearnFree.org – a program of Goodwill Community Foundation® and Goodwill Industries of Eastern NC Inc.® (GIENC®),

"Simply put, an app is a type of software that allows you to perform specific tasks. Applications for desktop or laptop computers are sometimes called desktop applications, while those for mobile devices are called mobile apps."

During an internet search, I found that NephCure which provides "detailed information about the diseases that cause Nephrotic Syndrome (NS) and Focal Segmental Glomerulosclerosis (FSGS)" (and was one of the first organizations to interview me about CKD, by the way) –

was way ahead of me in discussing apps. This is what's on their website:

Diet and Nutrition Apps

- KidneyAPPetite – Gives daily summaries of key nutrients for kidney health, check the nutritional value of foods before you eat it, and provides printable summaries to refer to. Great for patients on a renal diet! *Cost: Free, Device: iOS*

- Pocket Dietitian – Created by a Nephrologist, allows you to choose your health conditions and dietary restrictions to see recommended foods as well as keep track of what you have eaten. You can even see your past nutrition in graph form. *Cost: Free, Device: iOS and Android*

- My Food Coach – is designed to help you understand and manage all of your nutritional requirements. This app offers personalized nutrition information, recipes and meal plans. *Cost: Free, Device: iOS and Android*

- HealthyOut – Enables you to search and order nearby healthy food and browse for healthy options while out to eat. You can even choose a specific diet such as gluten free! *Cost: Free, Device: iOS and Android*

- Restaurant Nutrition – Allows you to search restaurants and look at nutritional values, locate

nearby restaurants, and keep a food journal. The Restaurant Nutrition application shows
nutritional information of restaurant
foods. *Cost: Free, Device: iOS and Android*

While I could easily go to most of the apps' websites by clicking on the name while I held down the control button (in the digital version of this book), this was not the case with Pocket Dietician. I was able to find it and lots of descriptive information about it in the Google Play store, but kept getting the message that I had no devices. The help function on the site was not helpful.

I have KidneyAPPetite on my phone, but keep using KidneyDiet instead. It keeps track of the 3 Ps (protein, potassium, and the one missing from food labels: phosphorous), sodium, calories, carbohydrates, cholesterol, and fat, and fluid intake. The very nice part of the app? You can add the foods you eat that are not on the food list provided. Unfortunately, this is the one I mentioned in the first paragraph. This is what's presently on their website:

The KidneyDiet® app is no longer being sold or supported. It, and all your data, will continue to reside on your device unless you delete it.

Thank you for your patronage. We hope KidneyDiet® has helped you.

Sincerely,
The KidneyDiet® Team

I consider this a great loss for those looking for a simple nutritional app for their CKD.

What about My Food Coach? It has an extra feature that my favorite lacked: a warning when a recipe would bring you over your renal diet limits. It's recipe oriented, which doesn't endear it to me since I like to experiment cooking my big five ounces of protein daily with my three different size servings of different fruits that are on my renal diet. I also avoid red meat.

HealthyOut, while not specifically for CKD, does have a function for the Mediterranean diet which is more often than not recommended for us. I thought this was a hoot since it never occurred to me that you can check restaurant foods by the restaurant name. I am adding this app to my iPhone.

Restaurant Nutrition is another app offered by Google Play, which means I can't even get into it. I did get through to the reviews and couldn't find any positive ones. I didn't see the point in pursuing this any further.

There are even kidney disease games, such as Kidney-Warrior, to teach yourself and your loved ones about your disease. This is the author's description of the game:

"A new hero emerges to fight a dreadful illness. A quest to save his father. A brand NEW approach to mobile gaming •Play as Glo, a young hero on his exciting adventure to save his father •SHOOT, SMACK, and SPIN your way through 3 different and exciting stages, packed with hours of gaming •LEARN about what kidneys do and how kidney disease affects people worldwide Created on behalf of Project ARK, an organization focused to support research efforts on combating kidney disease. As a high school organization, Project ARK seeks to raise awareness on campus and within the community."

To borrow a term from a now defunct cigarette brand: We've come a long way, baby!

10/31/16 *TED Doesn't Talk to Me; But YouTube Does*

After last week's accolades for the blog about apps for kidney disease, I thought I would keep on the electronic trail and jump right over to one of the big boys: TED Talks. I was both excited and a bit apprehensive since this is new territory for me. I have heard some of my children talk about them, but never explored these talks for myself.

What new information could I learn here? Would it be easier or harder to understand? And just what were T.E.D. Talks anyway? Doing what I like to do best, I jumped in for a bit of research.

This is directly from their website:

"TED is a nonpartisan nonprofit devoted to spreading ideas, usually in the form of short, powerful talks. TED began in 1984 as a conference where Technology, Entertainment and Design converged, and today covers almost all topics — from science to business to global issues — in more than 110 languages. Meanwhile, independently run TEDx events help share ideas in communities around the world.

Considering what's been going on with our other worldly politics this election, I thought I would check the meaning of nonpartisan just to make sure it had a meaning other than the one I'd been hearing bantered around. According to the Encarta Dictionary, it means "not belonging to, supporting, or biased in favor of a political party." I wasn't so sure that's what it meant for TED, so I used the synonym function in Word; that made much more sense: impartial, unaligned, unbiased, unprejudiced, neutral, and so on.

Now that we know what TED is, let's plunge right in and do some exploring. I searched Chronic Kidney Disease and got no hits. That's all right; a synonym is renal disease. I'll search that. All that came up was "Timothy Ihrig: What we can do to die well." That's not exactly what I was looking for.

I know, I'll type in kidney failure. Hmmm, that didn't work very well, either. I found two interesting talks, "Siddhartha Mukherjee: Soon we'll cure diseases with a cell, not a pill" and "Anthony Atala: Printing a human kidney," as well as two blogs that may have peripherally included CKD. No, these were not the talks about living with CKD that I'd hoped to find.

What other term could I search? I know, how about just-plain-kidney? I got three pages of hits which weren't really hits at all if you were looking for living with Chronic Kidney Disease. While TED Talks cover a variety of interesting topics, I don't think they're CKD specific right now. Maybe in the future...

I was a little crestfallen, but then I remembered that when I first decided to become a CKD Awareness Advocate and wrote *What Is It and How Did I Get It? Early Stage Chronic Kidney Disease*, I made a couple of

YouTubes as marketing devices. They were terrible, but did include some helpful information. When you've picked yourself up from the floor after getting your belly laughs at my expense (cringe), start exploring YouTube for CKD information by looking at the side bar on each of my woebegone entries into the world of YouTube. The list of videos continues and goes on and on. Yay!

Of course, just as when you're looking online - or choosing a book - or a blog to follow, you need to be careful to separate the wheat from the chaff. There are charlatans and scammers here, just as there are respected physicians and patients bravely sharing their stories.

But what is YouTube anyway? Their 'About" page tells us,

"Launched in May 2005, YouTube allows billions of people to discover, watch, and share originally-created videos. YouTube provides a forum for people to connect, inform, and inspire others across the globe and acts as a distribution platform for original content creators and advertisers large and small.

YouTube is a Google company."

You'll also find some YouTubes I posted that show friends, family, or me dancing either the Blues or East Coast Swing. My point? Anyone can post anything provided it does not include:

Nudity or sexual content

Violent or graphic content

Hateful content

Spam, misleading metadata, and scams

Harmful or dangerous content

Copyright (Me, here, this refers to copyrighted material.)

Threats

I chose one or two posts to see the quality we can find
here. I noticed one of the physicians I'd had content
with as an advocate, Dr. Robert Provenzano, posted
about the causes of CKD on 2/3/09 and it was highly
informative… but getting close to seven years old.

I wanted something more recent and found it. This one
by Danuta Trzebinska, MD, of US San Diego Health deals
with possible symptoms of CKD and was posted last
year.

But then I found YouTube about kidney cleanses which
could be harmful to already damaged kidneys. Dr. Josh
Axe was not particularly targeting CKD patients, but as a
new CKD patient, how could you know that? Some of
the herbs he suggests are harmful to ALREADY COM-
PROMISED kidneys. You need to be careful about which
videos are for those with CKD and which are for those

without CKD. Of course, you're checking everything you see with your nephrologist before you act on it. Right? You are, aren't you? You've got to protect your kidneys, so please (Let's make that pretty please.) do.

I'm wondering what other electronic helps I could explore. We've looked at apps, TED Talks, and YouTube. What other electronic aids do you know about that I don't? I'll be more than happy to explore it for myself which means I'll be exploring it for you, too, since it's going to end up being the next blog.

Today is Halloween. You know those treats? Why not treat yourself by not eating them? It's hard, but it can be done.

11/7/16 *Starting My Day*

Every day, I spend the morning doing 'kidney work' as I call it. That means looking for Chronic Kidney Disease related articles on Facebook, Twitter, LinkedIn, Instagram, Pinterest, and perusing the various medical newsletters to which I've subscribed. This takes a minimum of two hours. I also post something on most of these sites as *SlowItDownCKD*.

I noticed I'd been reading more and more about the plant based diet being good for CKD patients, so that's what I posted on *SlowItDownCKD*'s Facebook page on November 1. Then I started receiving emails from readers about it.

One was a very interesting, but undocumented, chart concerning how avoiding red meat lowers the risk of CKD. There was no title … and to make it worse, the reader couldn't remember where she found it. She was frustrated; I was frustrated. So I did a little digging.

I started with a site that's fast becoming one of my favorites – NephJC, a journal club. According to their website,

"It is the teaching session where trainees and teachers exchange roles. Journal Club is the area where the flipped classroom has been fully implemented in medical education. Read and study the article at home, and then use classroom time to critically debate the methods, results and interpretation of the article."

As both a former high school and college instructor, I can tell you this method of teaching seemed to have sparked some super creative thoughts in my classroom.

This reader also mentioned that she lost so much weight – without being hungry – on the plant based diet that her nephrologist asked her to gain weight so that she wouldn't "be at the bottom of BMI or below." You know this grabbed my attention.

At the same time we were corresponding, another CKD Awareness Advocate posted in a private FB group (Hence, the reason he remains unnamed.) that in his last two nephrology labs, he raised his GFR something like eight or nine points and had nothing to attribute it to but changing to a plant based diet.

As a reminder, here's the definition of GFR from *What Is It and How Did I Get It? Early Stage Chronic Kidney Disease:*

"Glomerular filtration rate [if there is a lower case "e" before the term, it means estimated glomerular filtration rate] which determines both the stage of kidney disease and how well the kidneys are functioning."

Let's look at this a little more closely. In *The Book of Blogs: Moderate Stage Chronic Kidney Disease, Part 2*, I wrote a blog about the limited history of nephrology and included mention of the five stages of CKD. Basically, the higher your GFR, the better your kidneys are working. So this means the other advocate's kidneys are functioning better now that he's on a plant based diet. Why?

I turned to Dr. Greger's NutritionFacts.org on YouTube for a better explanation than any I could offer. Dr. Greger is Michael Greger, described on Nutrition-Facts.org as:

"a physician, New York Times bestselling author, and internationally recognized speaker on nutrition, food safety, and public health issues. A founding member and Fellow of the American College of Lifestyle Medicine, Dr. Greger is licensed as a general practitioner specializing in clinical nutrition. He is a graduate of the Cornell University School of Agriculture and Tufts University School of Medicine."

NutritionFacts.org, while new to me, describes itself on its site as:

"a strictly non-commercial, science-based public service provided by Dr. Michael Greger, providing free updates on the latest in nutrition research via bite-sized videos. There are more than a thousand videos on nearly every aspect of healthy eating, with new videos and articles uploaded every day."

I thoroughly enjoyed his analogy of overloading the kidneys with meat protein to that of constantly revving a car's engine, especially since that's the same analogy I used in my first CKD book. He also mentions inflammation as a contributing cause of lower GFR. I'm glad I've discovered his website and intend to take a closer look at it…just not now.

Now I'm really interested in going back to that reader comment about losing weight on the plant based diet. I wanted to know – what else? – why. I spent most of yesterday researching. The consensus seems to be that not having to count calories or portion control may have something to do with it. Then again, maybe it's the lack of cookies, cakes, and candies. The few medical studies I did find were far too complicated for me to understand, much less explain. Are there any readers out there who can help? I have one particular reader in mind and hope that she will immediately respond.

Let's see if I can do any better with finding out why the nephrologist of the reader I'm corresponding with doesn't want her to "be at the bottom of BMI or below." Aha! A study by US National Library of Medicine National Institutes of Health suggests that "that combined effects of low BMI … and serum albumin level … are associated with CKD progression."

Maybe we should take a look at "serum albumin level." Serum means it's the clear part of your blood, the part without red or white blood cells. This much is fairly common knowledge. Albumin is not. Medlineplus, part of The National Institutes of Health's U.S. National Library of Medicine tells us, "Albumin is a protein made by the liver. A serum albumin test measures the amount of this protein in the clear liquid portion of the blood."

Uh-oh, this is also not good: a high level of serum albumin indicates progression of your kidney disease. Conversely, kidney disease can cause a high level of serum albumin.

Even with yesterday's research, this blog has taken quite a while to complete … and not just because I was doing the wash while I wrote it, or because I was enjoying having the window to my right open as I wrote. I can see this becoming several additional blogs… if there's reader interest.

11/14/16 *A Change is Gonna Come... Or is It?*

This has been a confusing week here in the United
States. You see, we have a new president-elect. I'm not
going to deal with politics in today's blog, but rather
some of the fears we have concerning our health care
under this new president. We are Chronic Kidney Disease patients and we have heard so many conflicting
rumors.

Let's start off with a little reassurance in this confusing
time. CBS's Lesley Stahl interviewed President-elect
Donald Trump on *60 Minutes* yesterday.

For those of us who might need some background, CBS
is the Columbia Broadcasting System which, of course
(It is 2016, after all.), now includes videos as well as live
television. You can also find them on YouTube via the
specific show's title.

According to IMDb (which describes itself as "...the
world's most popular and authoritative source for mov-
ie, TV and celebrity content....") *60 Minutes* is:

"The oldest and most-watched newsmagazine on television gets the real story on America's most prevalent
issues. CBS News correspondents contribute segments
to each hour long episode....."

And who is Lesley Stahl? Bio.com tells us, "Lesley Stahl
is an award-winning television journalist. She's served
as co-editor of *60 Minutes* and anchored the news pro-

gram *48 Hours Investigates*." These are not my usual sources, nor is this my usual sort of blog. However, it's the necessary blog today.

Following is the segment of her interview with the president elect about Obamacare which you may know as the Affordable Care Act (ACA).

"Lesley Stahl: Let me ask you about Obamacare, which you say you're going to repeal and replace. When you replace it, are you going to make sure that people with pre-conditions are still covered?

Donald Trump: Yes. Because it happens to be one of the strongest assets.

Stahl: You're going to keep that?

Trump: Also, with the children living with their parents for an extended period, we're gonna–

Stahl: You're gonna keep that–

Trump: Very much try and keep that. Adds cost, but it's very much something we're going to try and keep.

Stahl: And there's going to be a period if you repeal it and before you replace it, when millions of people could lose — no?

Trump: No, we're going to do it simultaneously. It'll be just fine. We're not going to have, like, a two-day period and we're not going to have a two-year period where there's nothing. It will be repealed and replaced. And we'll know. And it'll be great healthcare for much less money. So it'll be better healthcare, much better, for less money. Not a bad combination."

Is he definitive? Is he absolute? No, but what makes this hopeful is that during his campaign he announced, "On day one of the Trump Administration, we will ask Congress to immediately deliver a full repeal of Obamacare." Thank you to Trump's campaign website for this quote. We can see the softening of that position that we need.

We have pre-existing conditions. We cannot abide with a presidency that doesn't support healthcare which allows for this. I did say this would be a non-political blog, so no more adamancy from me... if I can help it.

What does the president elect say about Medicare? Those of us over 65 (That's me.) have Medicare as our primary insurance. I am lucky enough to have a secondary insurance through my union. How many of the rest of us are? By the way, if Medicare doesn't pay, neither does my secondary.

Here's what Trump had to say in a rally in Iowa on December 11th of last year:

"So, you've been paying into Social Security and Medicare...but we are not going to cut your Social Security and we're not cutting your Medicare...."

A little clarification is in order. According to their web-site at Medicare.gov, "Medicare is the federal health insurance program for people who are 65 or older, certain younger people with disabilities, and people with End-Stage Renal Disease (permanent kidney failure requiring dialysis or a transplant, sometimes called ESRD)..."

"Medicaid is a joint federal and state program that helps with medical costs for some people with limited income and resources. Medicaid also offers benefits not normally covered by Medicare, like nursing home care and personal care services," according to their website at Medicare.gov.

But then I found the following in a Forbes article by Janet Novack on 11/10/16.

"... two big spending cuts Trump has endorsed— a House Republican plan to cut Medicaid spending by $500 billion over a decade by turning it into a capped 'block grant' payment to the states and the 'penny a year' plan, which requires that all non-defense, discretionary spending be cut 1% a year in nominal terms, saving $750 billion over a decade (without, conveniently, spelling out which programs would get chopped)."

I admit it. I am in over my head. Does this mean that while Medicare will pay if you have ESRD, you still may be on the hook for personal care services IF Trump's capped block grant payment to states comes into being? Does it mean dialysis will be covered, but possibly not a nursing home stay necessitated by something secondary to your dialysis?

I don't have ESRD, but Medicare (and my secondary insurance) covers my labs and nephrologist's appointments. Let's say the cap goes through, I have a UTI – heaven forbid – that causes me to need a nurse (I know, I'm stretching the issue.), but my income has gone way down. Will Medicaid be available?

While I meant to write a reassuring blog today, I think I've raised more issues to question instead. I am not a politician, nor am I politically savvy. BUT, I am a Chronic Kidney Disease patient who needs some kind of reassurance that I won't be left without the coverage I need.

Hey, that's another thing: whatever happened to Trump's campaign promise about letting us order less expensive medications from other countries? Did I miss the update on that one?

11/21/16 *Clean...or Dirty?*

My daughter brought a friend to a party we were both attending a few weeks ago. We all enjoyed each other so we talked about the possibility of going out to dinner together at some future date. Being well aware of my renal restrictions and how that sometimes limits our choice of restaurants, I asked my daughter's friend how he likes to eat. He said, "Clean."

I've heard this before, as you probably have, too. Yet, I wasn't sure exactly what it meant. And that's why I'm researching it today and seeing just how it does – or doesn't – fit into our usual renal diet. Will someone get the dictionary, please? Thanks.

According to my personal favorite, The Merriam-Webster, clean means

: free from dirt, marks, etc.

: not dirty

: tending to keep clean

: free from pollution or other dangerous substances

Maybe it's that last definition that applies to eating? Hmmm, I need to take a closer look at this.

In her nutrition blog on another of my favorites – The MayoClinic – this past summer, Katherine Zeratsky,

R.D., L.D., suggested these as the main tenets of clean eating:

- Eat more real foods. Sound familiar? One of the tenets of the Mayo Clinic Diet is eating more real foods and fewer processed or refined foods. Convenience food is OK, sometimes even necessary, just make sure that what's in that can or package is the real thing with few other ingredients.

- Eat for nourishment. Eat regular, balanced meals and healthy snacks that are nourishing and not too rushed. Eat at home more often and prepare food in healthy ways. Pack food to eat away from home when on the road, at work or activities. When you do eat out, choose wisely.

- Eat safe food. This is my addition to the idea of clean eating. Based on the name itself, clean food should be safe. Practice food safety by washing produce before consumption (you may consider buying organic as well), keeping raw meats separate from produce from the grocery store to home, cooking food to proper temperatures and chilling food quickly after service.

By the way, R.D. means Registered Dietician and L.D. is Licensed Dietitian. Most states require at least one of these in order for the person to provide nutrition or diet advice.

This sounds too simple. Let's look a bit more. I found loads of articles on sites I didn't recognize by people I hadn't heard of, so I decided to take a look at a site specifically for clean eaters. This is from Clean Eating Magazine.

"The soul of eating clean is consuming food the way nature delivered it, or as close to it as possible. It is not a diet; it's a lifestyle approach to food and its preparation, leading to an improved life – one meal at a time.

Eat five to six times a day - Three meals and two to three small snacks. Include a lean protein, plenty of fresh fruit and vegetables, and a complex carbohydrate with each meal. The steady intake of clean food keeps your body energized and burning calories efficiently all day long.

Choose organic clean foods whenever possible.

Drink at least two liters of water a day.

Limit your alcohol intake to one glass of antioxidant-rich red wine a day.

Get label savvy - Clean foods contain just one or two ingredients. Any product with a long ingredient list is human-made and not considered part of a clean diet.

Avoid processed and refined foods - This includes white flour, sugar, bread and pasta. Enjoy complex carbs such as whole grains instead.

Steer clear of anything high in trans fats, anything fried or anything high in sugar. Avoid preservatives, color additives and toxic binders, stabilizers, emulsifiers and fat replacers.

Consume healthy fats.

Aim to have essential fatty acids, or EFAs, incorporated into your clean diet every day.

Learn about portion sizes - Work towards eating within them. When eating clean, diet is as much about quantity as it is quality."

Wow! And there's much more on their site.

There are just a few things that concern me here, specifically about the contents of those three meals and two to three small snacks. How can I stretch my five ounces of protein over all these meals and snacks? And my three servings each of only certain fruits and vegetables? I suppose I could skip the protein on one of them and have only one ounce at each of the others.

Do you know what one ounce of protein looks like? One egg, ¼ tablespoon of peanut better, or 2 bites of meat (although I don't eat red meat), poultry, or seafood. That last one is subjective; I just used the scale to test it out. I imagine it could be different if your mouth is smaller or larger than mine. I also didn't take into account the foods not on the renal diet, such as beans and nuts.

I'm attempting to avoid carbohydrates as much as I can in order to lose some weight, but my renal diet allows for 7 or 8 choices of these a day and 3 of fruits – which I do eat in moderation. There may be a problem with the whole grains recommended for clean eating since whole grains are high in phosphorous, something Chronic Kidney Disease patients need to watch. Chapter 8 of *What Is It and How Did I Get It? Early Stage Chronic Kidney Disease* explains the renal diet I follow in detail.

Other than those objections, I like the sound of clean eating. However, I do remember going to a clean eating restaurant when they first started opening and finding I was severely limited as to what I could order. Yep, whole grains, fruits and vegetables not on my diet, and too much protein. I checked out the vegetarian dishes, but found them huge. Funny to think of that as a negative, isn't it?

As usual, it looks like this is something you have to decide for yourself according to your renal diet since each of us is different. Would I try a clean eating restaurant again? Sure. Would I try clean eating at home? Maybe, although the whole grains thing bothers me.

11/28/16 *Cleaning Out*

Today I get to finish the final edits for my novel **Portal in Time** and submit it to my publisher. That means the next step is cleaning out my files and my computer. Writers accumulate an awful lot of unnecessary material when researching for a book.

That simple thought got me to thinking about another kind of cleaning out, the body kind. By the way, it seems the words cleanse and detox – short for detoxification – are being used interchangeably. Whichever term we use, are they safe for us as Chronic Kidney Disease patients?

But first – there's always a first, isn't there? – a warning: if you're thinking of doing one for weight loss, don't. According to Medicine.Net,

"There is no scientific evidence that "detox" (short for detoxification) or "cleanse" diets result in rapid weight loss or have any health benefits, says Heather Mangieri, RDN, LDN, a spokeswoman for the Academy of Nutrition and Dietetics and founder of NutritionCheckUp in Pittsburgh.

Indeed, the opposite may be true: One study published in 2011 in the journal *Obesity* found that beginning a weight-loss diet with a fast or cleanse could be counterproductive."

Now wait just a minute, if they provide no "rapid weight loss or have any health benefits," why do people go to the trouble of doing them? I wrote about this just a bit in relation to brain fog in *SlowItDownCKD 2015*.

"...with CKD I'd talk over detoxing and/or taking supplements to support cell power with my nephrologist before actually following that advice. Some nephrologists are dead (Yikes! Wrong word choice) set against detoxifying while others have a more eclectic approach to gentle detoxifying."

Ah, so there MAY be some benefits in relation to brain fog. What's brain fog again? *The Book of Blogs: Moderate Stage Chronic Kidney Disease, Part 2* (I have got to get around to shortening that title.) can help us out here.

"According to integrative medicine expert Dr. Isaac Eliaz, when experiencing brain fog

'...people feel as if there is a thick fog dampening their mind. While the medical and mental health establishments don't generally recognize brain fog as a condition, it's a surprisingly common affliction that affects people of all ages. Symptoms include pervasive absentmindedness, muddled thought processes, poor memory recall, difficulty processing information, disorientation, fatigue, and others.'"

Well, what exactly is a detox? The Free Dictionary's medical dictionary offers this as one of its definitions:

"A short-term health regimen involving procedures thought to remove toxins from the body, such as drinking large amounts of liquid, eating a restricted diet or fasting, taking nutritional supplements, and undergoing enemas."

Now we get to the meat of the matter. Why do Chronic Kidney Disease patients need to be so careful about cleanses? I looked at the ingredient list of several different cleanses. The first product was Super Colon Cleanse. One of the first ingredients was Psyllium Husk Powder 1 g. Uh-oh. Not good for us. As Metamucil Advisor – the manufacturer of fiber products explains,

"Psyllium husk is a natural fiber that comes from the plant called Plantago Ovata. Plantago Ovata produces thousands of seeds that are coated with a gel like substance that is extracted to create psyllium husk. The psyllium husk is a natural soluble fiber laxative that can be consumed to add bulk to the feces. Consuming psyllium powder will draw water to the stool making it easier to have a bowl movement. Psyllium husk is recommended to not be taken by individuals who have kidney disease because it is high in magnesium that individuals with chronic kidney disease must avoid. It is highly recommended to consult your physician before starting any product of psyllium husk to make sure it is safe with any health conditions you might have."

Well, that's only one cleanse. Let's take a look at another. Dr. Tobias Colon: 14 Day Quick Cleanse is composed of herbs, no psyllium. But there's a problem there, too. As Chronic Kidney Disease patients we are cautioned against taking herbs, not so much because they will cause damage, but because we don't know how much of each is safe for our kidneys.

I thought I remembered writing about this in *What Is It and How Did I Get It? Early Stage Chronic Kidney Disease* – another really long title – and decided to find that information. Here it is:

"While none of this is established, the following might be toxic to the kidneys -wormwood, periwinkle, sassafras (I remember drinking sassafras tea as a child. Did that have any effect on my kidneys?) and horse chestnut just to name a few. Then there are the herbal supplements that might be harmful to CKD patients: alfalfa, aloe, bayberry, capsicum, dandelion, ginger, ginseng, licorice, rhubarb and senna. There are others, but they seemed too esoteric to include…."

Three is usually the magic number, so let's look at another product. This time at something labeled 'detox.' Baetea 14 Day Teatox is the one I chose. I think I liked the play on words: detox, teatox, a tea to detox. Lots of herbs, but then I looked at the last ingredient - Garcinia Cambogia. That rang a caution bell in my mind so I went right to a site about the side effects of this product.

"Our kidneys and liver remove toxins, waste and other substances from our body. They are the main organs designed to clean the body of impurities. People who already have diseases of the kidneys or liver should not take Garcinia Cambogia because their bodies might not be able to utilize and remove the supplement effectively."

sigh It looks like we'll just have to detox the old fashioned way, with increased fiber, as much water as your nephrologist permits, and exercise.

12/5/16 *Medical Individuals*

We all know I write about Chronic Kidney Disease, or CKD, but just what is that? When I wrote *What Is It and How Did I Get It? Early Stage Chronic Kidney Disease* six years ago, I defined CKD as "Damage to the kidneys for more than three months, which cannot be reversed but may be slowed." Although I'm not so sure about that "cannot be reversed" any more, this is simple, right?

Well, not exactly. Over the years, many readers have pointed out that they have another form of kidney disease. According to University Kidney Research Organization (UKRO), these are all considered kidney disease:

- Alport Syndrome

- Diabetic Nephropathy

- Fabry Disease

- Focal Segmental Glomerulosclerosis

- Glomerulonephritis

- IgA Nephropathy (Berger's Disease)

- Kidney Stones

- Minimal Change Disease

- Nephrotic Syndrome

- Polycystic Kidney Disease or PKD

Wait a minute. Chronic means of long duration. Then with the exception (hopefully) of kidney stones, these diseases can all be classified as CKD... but are they when it comes to treatment?

Dr. Joel Topf is a nephrologist who writes a blog of his own (Precious Bodily Fluids) and is a member of the eAJKD Advisory Board at American Journal of Kidney Disease. He must make great use of his time because he has helped develop teaching games for nephrology students and has written medical works. (Yeah, I'm impressed with him, too.)

He's also a Twitter friend. He contacted me the other day about an article in the *Clinical Journal of the American Society of Nephrology* entitled "The CKD Classification System in the Precision Medicine Era," which was written by Yoshio N. Hall and Jonathan Himmelfarb. You can read it for yourself on their site, but you'll need to join it and get yourself a user name and password. I didn't. Joel sent me the copy I needed.

My first reaction to his request was, "Sure!" Then I read the article and wondered if I could handle all the medicalese in it. Several readings later, I see why he asked me to write about it.

I say I have CKD stage 3B. You understand what I mean. So does my nephrologist. That's due to the KDOQI. As I explained in *The Book of Blogs: Moderate Stage Chron-*

ic Kidney Disease, Part 2, this is *The National Kidney Foundation Kidney Disease Out- Comes Quality Initiative* which was not put into place until 1997 and then updated only five years later in 2002. It introduced stages and put CKD on the world medical map. By the way, the 2012 revised guidelines helped raised awareness of CKD according to the CJASN article: "…from 4.7% to 9.2% among persons with CKD stages 3 and 4 in the United States …."

But something is missing. How can my stage 3 CKD be the same for someone who has, say, Nephrotic Syndrome? We may have the same GFR, but are our symptoms the same? Is the progression of our illnesses the same? What about our treatment? Our other test results?

Whoops! A certain someone looking over my shoulder as I type reminded me I need to define GFR. I especially like Medline Plus's definition that I used in *SlowItDownCKD 2015*:

"Glomerular filtration rate (GFR) is a test used to check how well the kidneys are working. Specifically, it estimates how much blood passes through the glomeruli each minute. Glomeruli are the tiny filters in the kidneys that filter waste from the blood."

I know, I know, I didn't explain what "the Precision Medicine Era" is, either. According to the article, "The underlying concept behind the Precision Medicine Initiative is that disease prevention and treatment strategies must take individual variability into account." Actually, President Obama first used the term in his State of the Union Address last year.

Alrighty now, back to why CKD staging is not necessarily precision medicine. It seems to center on one phrase – individual variability. I was diagnosed at age 60. I'm now almost 70. Where is the age adjustment in my treatment plan? Is there one? What about when I'm 80? 90? We know the body reacts differently to medications as we age. Is my nephrologist taking this into account? Is yours? I'm taking liberties with the definition of individual here; I don't think the authors meant within the individual, but rather amongst individuals.

I check my husband's blood test results for his GFR. FOR HIS AGE, he does not have CKD. But here's another point I've been ranting about that's brought up in this article. Many elders (Oh my! We're in that category already.) are not being told if they have stage 1 or stage 2 CKD because their doctors age adjust and so don't consider the results CKD. We're getting a little esoteric here. Is CKD really CKD if you've age adjusted your GFR readings?

My brain is starting to hurt and I haven't even written about the different diseases yet, although I did allude to them earlier. What impressed me most in this article is this (in discussing four different hypothetical patients): "Each would be classified as having stage 3 CKD with approximately the same eGFR, but it is patently obvious that virtually every aspect of clinical decision making ... would greatly differ in caring for these four individuals."

I have to agree in my layman way. I'm not a doctor, but I know that if you have Polycystic Kidney Disease and I don't, although our GFR is the same, I cannot receive the same treatment you do and you cannot receive the same treatment I do. Yes, they're both kidney diseases and both chronic, but they are not the same disease despite our having the same GFR.

There is no one size fits all here. Nor does there yet seem to be precision. My CKD at 70 is not the same as it was at 60. If I had diabetes, my CKD treatment would be different, too. I do have hypertension and that has already changed my CKD treatment.

This got me to thinking. How would every nephrologist find the time for this individualized treatment for each CKD patient? And what other tests will each patient need to determine treatment based on his/her UNIQUE form of CKD?

Thanks for the suggestion, Dr. Topf. This was worth writing about.

12/12/16 *Never Too Old to Learn*

Last week, we were delighted to have an overnight guest we hadn't seen for a year or two. While we were all waking ourselves up the next morning, I asked him if he'd like some coffee. Yep, he's my family; that look of delight on his face when he thought of coffee confirmed it.

Then I asked if he took milk in his coffee. Hmmm, more confirmation: he passed on the milk claiming lactose intolerance, another family trait. But when we got to the sugar question, he startled me. His response was something like no thanks, I have high cholesterol. After a moment of stunned silence, I asked why he connected cholesterol and sugar. He said his doctor told him to cut down on sugars to lower his cholesterol. Hmmm, very interesting.

This is the definition of cholesterol from *What Is It and How Did I Get It? Early Stage Chronic Early Disease*: "While the basis for both sex hormones and bile can cause blockages if it accumulates in the lining of a blood vessel."

If that doesn't ring a bell, here's the definition of dyslipidemia: "Abnormal levels of cholesterol, triglyceride or both"

Now we know there's a normal and an abnormal level of cholesterol and that can't be good. Is that a big deal?

It is if you have Chronic Kidney Disease. Dr. Joseph Vas-salotti, one of leading nephrologists in the U.S., ex-plained it to reporter Jane Brody in an interview which is included in *The Book of Blogs: Moderate Stage Chronic Kidney Disease, Part 1*.

"Good control of blood sugar, blood pressure, choles-terol levels and body weight can delay the loss of kidney function."

I repeat, "...can delay the loss of kidney function." That has been your ultimate goal since you were diagnosed, hasn't it?

You may become confused by the three different kinds of cholesterol readings when you see the results of your blood tests. I know I was, so I researched them and then wrote about them in *The Book of Blogs: Moderate Stage Chronic Kidney Disease, Part 2*.

"HDL is High Density Lipoprotein, the cholesterol that keeps your arteries clear or – as it's commonly called – the good cholesterol. LDL is Low Density Lipoprotein or the 'bad' kind that can clog your arteries. VLDL is Very Low Density Lipoprotein and one of the bad guys, too. It contains more triglycerides than protein and is big on clogging those arteries."

Wait a minute. Where did triglycerides come into this? According to the Mayo Clinic, "Triglycerides and choles-terol are separate types of lipids that circulate in your blood. Triglycerides store unused calories and provide your body with energy, and cholesterol is used to build cells and certain hormones. Because triglycerides and cholesterol can't dissolve in blood, they circulate throughout your body with the help of proteins that transport the lipids (lipoproteins)."

Still with me? Good, because you can do something about this. Sometimes, it's as simple as lifestyle changes like adjusting your diet. While I don't agree with all of this advice, it can get you started.

- *Avoid foods high in saturated fat and cholesterol such as whole milk, cheese and fat from meat.*

- *Bake, grill, broil and roast your poultry, fish and meat. Choose lean cuts of meat and trim off any fat.*

- *Eggs are an excellent source of protein, but the yolks are high in cholesterol. Try egg substitutes like Egg Beaters® or Scramblers®, or substitute two egg whites for a whole egg.*

- *Eat at least two servings of fish every week. Salmon, tuna, herring and trout contain good amounts of omega-3 fatty acids that lower your risk of heart disease.*

- *Try spreads like Benecol® or Take Control® in place of butter or margarine. Plant sterols and stanols in these spreads help lower cholesterol levels.*

- *Choose oils that are high in mono- and polyunsaturated fats: canola, olive, peanut, corn, safflower, soybean and sunflower.*

- *Read food labels and try to eliminate foods with trans-fats (found in hydrogenated oils, margarine and many commercially prepared snack foods).*

- *Eat kidney-friendly fruits and vegetables.*

Of course, if you're diabetic or prediabetic, you need to modify these suggestions for your diet.

As was suggested in this Everyday Health article included in *SlowItDownCKD 2015*, exercise will help.

Try these exercise options to help shed pounds and manage high cholesterol:

- *Walking*

- *Jogging or running*

- *Swimming*

- *Taking an aerobics class*

- *Biking*

- *Playing tennis, basketball, or other sports*

- *Using weight machines or lifting free weights to build muscle tone*

If life style changes don't work for you, your doctor may prescribe a statin. The Merriam-Webster Dictionary defines this as, "any of a group of drugs (as lovastatin and simvastatin) that inhibit the synthesis of cholesterol and promote the production of LDL-binding receptors in the liver resulting in a usually marked decrease in the level of LDL and a modest increase in the level of HDL circulating in blood plasma"

There are substantial arguments against taking statins, but there are also substantial arguments for taking them. This is something you have to discuss with your doctors since you have a unique medical condition.

Finally, sugar. What did my cousin's doctor mean about sugar's role in lowering his cholesterol? This was news to me, so I researched. Sure enough, my cousin's doctor was right. According to Progressive Health:

"Sugar is a good example of a carbohydrate with high glycemic index. It can, therefore, increase the amount of small, dense LDL particles in the blood.

Although health experts used to advocate that we cut the amount of sugar we consume because high blood sugar can cause insulin resistance and increase the risk of diabetes, there is now another reason to cut down on our sugar consumption.

A number of studies show that sugar can affect the kind and amount of cholesterol released into the blood."

So? According to the US National Library of Medicine National Institutes of Health, "...patients with pre-dialysis CKD appear to be more likely to die of heart disease than of kidney disease. CKD accelerates coronary artery atherosclerosis by several mechanisms, notably hypertension and dyslipidemia, both of which are known risk factors for coronary artery disease."

That's a pretty big 'so.'

12/19/16 *It's a Miracle!*

It's that time of year again... the time to believe in miracles. There's the miracle of Mary's virgin birth at Christmas. And there's the miracle of the Chanukah oil burning for eight nights instead of the one it was meant to. That got me to thinking about miracles and so, we have a different kind of several part blog beginning today. Consider it my gift to you this holiday season.

Miracles happen every day, too. We just need to take action to make them happen... and that's what I'd like to see us do with Chronic Kidney Disease by sharing the available information. This particular miracle is helping to alleviate the fear of needing dialysis and/or transplantation. This particular miracle is helping patients help themselves and each other. This particular miracle is helping doctors appreciate involved patients.

Yet, causing this miracle by sharing information is overlooked again and again. Chronic Kidney Disease, or CKD, is easily diagnosed by simple blood tests and urine tests (as we know), but who's going to take them if they have no idea the disease exists, is widespread, and may be lethal? By sharing information, those at high risk will be tested. Those already in the throes of CKD can be monitored and treated when necessary. While CKD is not curable, we know it is possible to slow down the progression of the decline in your kidney function.

According to the National Institutes of Health, "2014: Worldwide, an estimated 200 million people have chronic kidney disease (CKD)."

Before I was diagnosed, I had never heard of this disease… and apparently I'd had it for quite some time. Why weren't people sharing information about this? Couldn't that have prevented my developing it? At the time of my diagnose nine years ago, I meant doctors. I don't anymore. Nor do I leave causing a miracle by sharing to others.

This is my life. I have had Chronic Kidney Disease for nine years. As a college instructor who taught Research Writing at the time of my diagnose, I researched, researched, and researched again, but the only person I was sharing my research with was the nephrologist who treated me and monitored my condition. I may have expected a miracle there, but I didn't get one. Why?

I got to thinking about that and realized he already knew what I told him. That's when it struck me that if I expected a miracle with CKD, I would have to start sharing this information with the people who need it: the ones who didn't know, the ones who had just been diagnosed and were terrified, and the families of those with CKD who didn't know they also might be at risk. I went so far as to bring CKD education to the Native American Communities in Arizona since Native Americans are at high risk. I had the information and had experts willing to come to the communities to share that information.

We all know this is a costly, lethal disease if not caught early and treated... and that it's not just the elderly who are at risk. One out of ten people worldwide has CKD, yet an overwhelming number of them are unaware they have it. We know CKD can be treated, just not the way those who don't have it might expect. A diet with restrictions on protein, potassium, phosphorous and sodium may be one aspect of that treatment. Exercise, adequate sleep, and avoiding stress are some of the other aspects. Some patients – like me – may have to take medication for their high blood pressure since that also affects kidney function. Imagine preventing a death with lifestyle changes. Now imagine EXPECTING the miracle of preventing that death by sharing this information. Powerful, isn't it?

We know the basic method of diagnosing CKD is via routine blood and urine tests. Yet, many people do not undergo these tests during doctor or clinic visits, so don't know they have Chronic Kidney Disease, much less start treating it.

This is where the miracle I expected in my life began for me. I started speaking with every doctor of any kind that I knew or that my doctors knew and asked them to share the information. They were already experiencing time constraints, but suggested I write a fact sheet and leave it in their waiting rooms since they agreed there's no reason to wait until a person is in kidney failure and needs dialysis or a transplant to continue living before diagnosing and dealing with the illness.

My passion about producing this miracle multiplied threefold from that point on. So much so that I went one better and wrote a book with the facts. I was convinced we would be able to cause a miracle by sharing information about this disease. My goal was clear: have everyone routinely tested.

Dr. Robert Provenzano, a leading nephrologist in the United States, succinctly summed up the problem worldwide.

"Chronic Kidney Disease is an epidemic in the world…. As other countries become Westernized, we find the incidence of Chronic Kidney Disease and end-stage renal failure increases. We see this in India, and in China. We see this everywhere. …"

We repeatedly see diabetes and hypertension cited as the two major causes of CKD. Does your neighbor know this? How about the fellow at the gas station? Ask them what Chronic Kidney Disease is. More often than not, you'll receive a blank look – one we can't afford if you keep the statistic at the beginning of this paper in mind. We can cause a miracle to change this.

Sharing can be the cause of that miracle… but that's not something we can leave to the other guy. We each ARE the other guy. More on this next week.

For now, Merry Christmas, Happy Chanukah, Happy Kwanzaa (somehow implicit in this holiday is the miracle of bringing people together), and every other holiday I've inadvertently missed or don't know about.

I just got word that *Portal in Time* – my first novel – is available on Amazon.com. Consider that as a holiday gift for those friends not interested in CKD. Of course, I just happen to have four CKD books on Amazon.com for those who might be interested in CKD. Be part of a miracle.

12/26/16 *Miracles Redux*

Welcome to the last blog of 2016. I find it hard to believe another year has passed, although I do acknowledge that I'm a bit slower and more content to stay in my office to write rather than run around town. It's a bit harder to maintain my body, although my mind is doing fine… as long as I don't have to remember too much at once, that is. Well, my knees may have something to say, but I try to keep them happy with daily exercise and the braces.

 I sincerely hope you enjoyed a joyous Christmas if you celebrate. And that you continue to enjoy Chanukah and Kwanzaa if you celebrate. We'll be leaving for the Trans-Siberian Orchestra concert as soon as I finish the blog… a gift from us to us and one of the kids for Christmas. On Wednesday, we'll have our Annual Chanukah Gathering. Our New York daughter will be with us since her Chanukah gift is a plane ticket. Being a two religion family, we celebrate both Chanukah and Christmas.

Before I get to more about creating a miracle, I am proud to announce that Healthline has named *SlowItDownCKD* one of The Best Kidney Disease Blogs of 2016. Talk about being surprised… and honored. Sort of a nice Christmas present, don't you think? I suppose I can consider the publication of my novel, **Portal in Time**, my Chanukah present. I didn't do too shabbily this year.

Okay, on to more about miracles – or Part 2 – as I promised last week.

If CKD were common knowledge, if those in high risk categories were aware of it, we might have a chance of preventing the disease in those who don't have it yet and/or slowing down the progression of the decline in kidney function of those who have been already diagnosed.

Exactly how can we do that? On the most basic level, there's the spoken word. It's not just the medical community that can talk about the disease. I can as a patient. You can, too, because you know me and I've told you about the disease (and/or you suffer from CKD yourself). This is most effective in areas of the world that do not have access to - or money for - doctors and treatment. This is where we can prevent more and more of the disease by preventing more and more hypertension and diabetes.

If I tell you what I know about curtailing sodium intake in high blood pressure and you tell me what you know about smoking as it contributes to hypertension, we've just shared two important aspects in the prevention of high blood pressure. If I tell you what I know about sugar in diabetes and you tell me what you know about carbohydrates and diabetes, we've just shared two important aspects in the prevention of diabetes. Then my husband starts sharing what he knows... and your third cousin once removed shares with her East Indian neighbor what her nephrologist told her... and your boss's secretary shares what his boyfriend learned at his CKD awareness meeting, you've got a lot more people aware of what needs to be done about CKD. Sometimes causing a miracle is played out by sharing with people. Think of the miracle this kind of communication on a daily basis can cause.

The people you speak to will share with those they know, those they know will share with others they know until many, many more people become aware of CKD – just as that long ago Clairol hair coloring ad demonstrated how telling someone who tells someone can go on ad infinitum. Simplistic? Yes, but it works...and that's part of living the life of causing a miracle in CKD.

Then there's the printed word. If people are aware of CKD books and newspapers, business and educational publications can alert their populations that the disease exists and is lethal, but may be prevented and/or slowed down. Most businesses have wellness components. What perfect vehicles to transform the world's awareness of CKD.

For example: my four Chronic Kidney Disease books are sold in 106 countries. I have 107,000 readers. This in itself is a miracle, not just for me but for everyone who is in some way connected to the disease. It is not uncommon for one community member to buy the book, then share it with everyone else in their social circle. If there's a library, the books can be ordered and then shared for free.

I also share my information via this blog. A doctor in a remote village in India prints and translates it to share with whichever patient has the bus fare to make it to the clinic. That patient brings the translation back to his family, friends, neighbors, and whoever else he thinks may be interested. This nephrologist's view is the same as mine: We both need to live a life causing a miracle in Chronic Kidney Disease Awareness by sharing information.

People who may not have known Chronic Kidney Disease exists now know via this sharing. Others who have undergone the simple blood and urine tests to diagnose the illness can share that the tests are not painful, other than the initial pinch of the needle for the blood draw. You would be surprised how many people, even in the high risk groups, don't take the tests because they fear there will be pain involved. No sharing, no awareness. No awareness, no diagnose. No diagnose, no slowing down the disease.

I've got some more thoughts, but we'll have to leave them for Part 3 in the New Year. This blog is getting too long and my family is waiting for me. Happy New Year to each and every one of you. Please be safe if you're going out to celebrate.

Index

My Notes:

Have you read my other Chronic Kidney Disease books? Available on Amazon.com and B&N.com

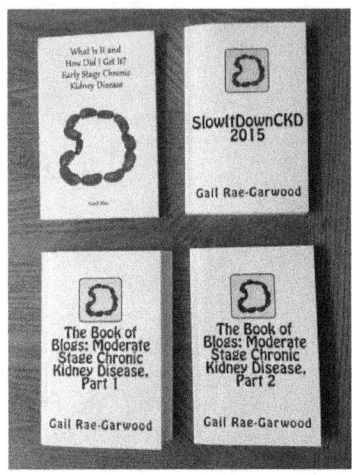

Follow the blog at

https://gailraegarwood.wordpress.com

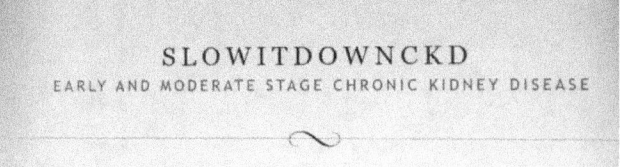

On Twitter, Instagram, and Pinterest, go to

@SlowItDownCKD

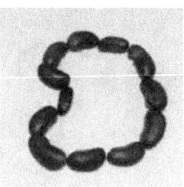

And then, there's the Facebook page at

https://www.facebook.com/

SlowItDownCKD/

On LinkedIn, you can find me at

Gail Rae-Garwood

Don't forget you can email me at

SlowItDownCKD@gmail.com

If you'd like to read a time travel romance

(Amazon.com and B&N.com)

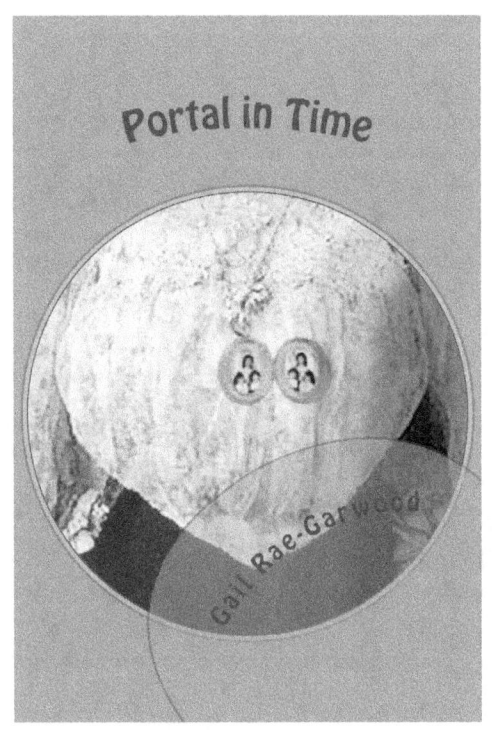